Cardiomyopathy - A Comprehensive Overview

Edited by Aleksandar Kibel

Published in London, United Kingdom

Cardiomyopathy - A Comprehensive Overview
http://dx.doi.org/10.5772/intechopen.1008627
Edited by Aleksandar Kibel

Contributors
Aleksandar Kibel, Andrew Ndakotsu, Angelina Borizanova, Dora Uršić, Eleanor E. Bashian, Elizabeth J. Bashian, Justin Chang, Keyur B. Shah, Mohammed Makkiya, Sultan Alotaibi, Valentina Robila, Ye In Christopher Kwon, Zubair A. Hashmi

First published in London, United Kingdom, 2026 by IntechOpen
IntechOpen is the global imprint of INTECHOPEN LIMITED, registered in England and Wales, registration number: 11086078, 167-169 Great Portland Street, London, W1W 5PF, United Kingdom

For EU product safety concerns: IN TECH d.o.o., Prolaz Marije Krucifikse Kozulić 3, 51000 Rijeka, Croatia, info@intechopen.com or visit our website at intechopen.com.

British Library Cataloguing-in-Publication Data
A catalogue record for this book is available from the British Library

Cardiomyopathy - A Comprehensive Overview
Edited by Aleksandar Kibel
p. cm.

This title is part of the Cardiology and Cardiovascular Medicine Book Series, Volume 17
Topic: Cardiovascular Diseases and Health
Series Editor: Kaan Kırali
Topic Editor: Mahi L. Ashwath

Print ISBN 978-1-83635-569-4
Online ISBN 978-1-83635-568-7
eBook (PDF) ISBN 978-1-83635-570-0
ISSN 3033-361X

If disposing of this product, please recycle the paper responsibly.

IntechOpen Book Series
Cardiology and Cardiovascular Medicine
Volume 17

Aims and Scope of the Series

Today, since molecular science on structural causes of oncological pathologies and their molecular treatments are developing at an unbelievable rate, the primary medical cause of death in the twenty-first century will be cardiovascular disease. Neither pandemics that threaten all humanity nor deterioration in the ecosystem will be able to change this fact. Especially, this century seems poised to witness an incredible struggle against atherosclerotic disease, which develops in the arterial walls and results in narrowing and occlusion of the arterial lumen. In addition to this disease, there has been an increasing prevalence of heart rhythm problems, deterioration of heart valves due to aging, and heart failure. Serious vascular pathologies such as stenosis and occlusion, dissection and rupture, and aneurysmal enlargement are also major concerns. Medical and invasive treatment methods may work to save human lives, but they will never provide a real solution. All kinds of medical, technological, and genetic engineering developments obtained in these processes have not yet been sufficient to alleviate or eliminate cardiovascular disease. This book series, Cardiology and Cardiovascular Medicine, includes three topics. The first, Cardiovascular Diseases and Health, reviews important cardiovascular diseases and the developments in their prognosis. The second topic, Cardiovascular Electrophysiology, illuminates the abnormal functioning of the cardiac conduction system, which is caused by all heart pathologies and negatively affects prognosis. The third topic in this series, Cardiovascular Surgery, details treatment for cardiovascular pathologies and how to regulate normal physiological functions with percutaneous or extracorporeal interventions.

Meet the Series Editor

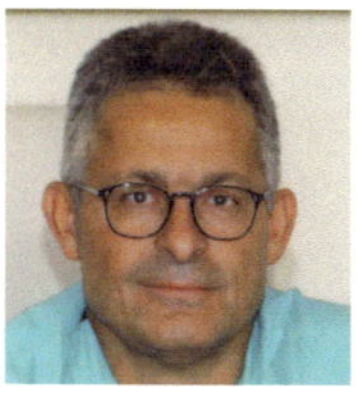

After completing his studies at the Medicine Faculty of Istanbul University in 1990, Prof. Kaan Kırali fulfilled his mandatory medical service and commenced his residency training at Koşuyolu Heart and Research Hospital in 1992. Following five years of assistant education, he pursued further training in England and the USA in 1998. Specializing in laparoscopic and minimally invasive cardiac surgery, he earned the titles of consultant cardiovascular surgeon in 1998, Assistant Professor in 1999, Associate Professor in 2002, and Chief in 2005 at the same hospital. Prof. Kırali also developed an interest in preventive medicine, obtaining an MSc in Public Health from Istanbul University in 2000. Over the past two decades, he has concentrated his scientific pursuits on cardiovascular repairs requiring specialized experience. With his expertise in coronary artery surgery, minimally invasive cardiac surgery, valve repair, and aortic root surgery, he has established new methods for awake coronary bypass revascularization, a new surgical approach for AVR during first and re-operations, aortic valve-sparing procedure, and radiofrequency ablation. Notably, he pioneered awake complete coronary artery bypass grafting (CABG) with bilateral internal mammary arteries (BIMA) and played a crucial role in advancing aortic root surgery with a new aortotomy incision, simplifying aortic valve interventions. Since the year 2000, Prof. Kırali has expanded his interests to heart transplantation, and in recent years, to left ventricular assist devices. He has served as the head of the transplantation department since 2015 and currently continues his work as the director of Koşuyolu High Specialization Education and Research Hospital in Istanbul, Turkey. In his prolific career, he has authored numerous papers in SCI journals, contributed to various book chapters, and served as an editor and reviewer for multiple academic journals. Additionally, he has edited several international books in the field of cardiovascular medicine.

Meet the Volume Editor

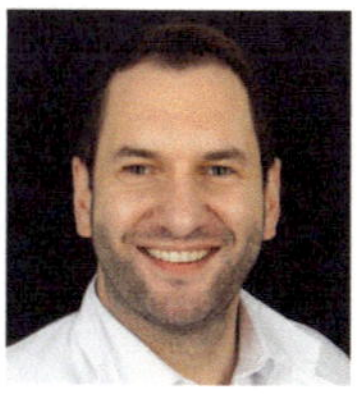

Dr. Aleksandar Kibel is an Associate Professor and subspecialist in Cardiology, currently serving as the Head of Internal Medicine and Cardiology at the International Medical Center Priora. A top-tier graduate with a perfect 5. 0 GPA, he earned his Ph.D. in 2014, focusing on cardiovascular physiology. With over a decade of experience at the Osijek University Hospital Center, he now leads the Scientific Unit for Medical Research and the MEFOS-2 research group within the Center of Excellence for Personalized Health Care. He is a Senior Research Associate in both basic and clinical medical sciences, having led multiple institutional projects (IP-8, IP-27) and participated in international training across the US, Europe, and Asia. A native speaker of Croatian and German, Dr. Kibel has served as the head of the Medical Program in German at the Faculty of Medicine in Osijek. He is a prolific author and editor, specifically noted for his work on the renin–angiotensin system, and serves as a mentor to five doctoral students.

Contents

Preface

Cardiomyopathies comprise a diverse group of myocardial diseases in which structural and/or functional abnormalities of the heart muscle cannot be explained solely by coronary artery disease, hypertension, valvular disease, or congenital disabilities. They range from primary disorders, often driven by genetic predisposition, inflammatory injury, immune dysregulation, or idiopathic processes, to secondary forms that arise in systemic conditions such as metabolic, infiltrative, toxic, or endocrine disease. Despite their heterogeneity, cardiomyopathies share a common clinical relevance: they are major contributors to heart failure, arrhythmias, thromboembolic complications, and sudden cardiac death, frequently affecting patients across a broad age spectrum and presenting with variable trajectories from subtle symptoms to advanced, life-threatening disease.

Over the past few decades, advances in imaging, molecular biology, and computational analysis have refined how cardiomyopathies are recognized and categorized. Echocardiography and cardiac magnetic resonance have enabled more precise characterization of phenotypes, revealing patterns of remodeling, fibrosis, edema, and infiltration that inform both prognosis and management. In parallel, genetic testing has illuminated pathways underlying hypertrophic, dilated, arrhythmogenic, and restrictive phenotypes, while enabling cascade screening and earlier identification of at-risk relatives. Yet cardiomyopathy remains, in many respects, a clinical syndrome rather than a single entity: similar phenotypes can arise from distinct mechanisms, and the same mechanism can manifest with different morphologic patterns depending on timing, comorbidities, and individual susceptibility.

At the core of cardiomyopathy lies an interplay between initiating insults and the heart's adaptive, and ultimately maladaptive, responses. Early triggers may involve sarcomeric dysfunction, cytoskeletal instability, mitochondrial impairment, microvascular dysregulation, autoimmune activation, or extracellular matrix perturbations. Once established, the disease frequently becomes self-sustaining through integrated circulatory and neurohormonal changes that reshape cardiac loading conditions and energetics. Myocyte injury and death, inflammatory signaling, and fibroblast activation converge on remodeling processes that may preserve cardiac output in the short term but gradually erode mechanical efficiency and electrical stability. Consequently, cardiomyopathy research increasingly focuses not only on "what starts the process," but also on "what maintains it"—the molecular, cellular, and tissue-level mechanisms that link initial injury to progressive dysfunction.

This volume, *Cardiomyopathy – A Comprehensive Overview*, is grounded in that evolving perspective. Rather than revisiting only the most familiar frameworks, it highlights mechanisms and forms of cardiomyopathy that may receive less attention in routine discussions, yet are increasingly recognized as clinically and biologically important. Several chapters address emerging scientific advances that deepen our understanding of pathophysiology, particularly the processes that sustain disease once remodeling has begun, as well as the mechanistic steps that govern initiation and progression.

A central theme is the contribution of immune mechanisms to primary cardiomyopathies, where inflammatory pathways can act as triggers, amplifiers, or modifiers of phenotype and outcome. The book also examines Takotsubo cardiomyopathy, a striking model of stress-related myocardial dysfunction that challenges traditional boundaries between functional disturbance and structural disease. In addition, infiltrative cardiomyopathies are explored as paradigms in which the myocardium is altered by abnormal deposition or cellular infiltration, often with subtle early findings but profound consequences as they advance. The complex myocardial response to aortic stenosis is considered, with emphasis on specific aspects of remodeling beyond the valve itself, highlighting the transition from compensatory hypertrophy to maladaptive fibrosis and dysfunction. Finally, atrial cardiomyopathies are discussed as an expanding concept that reframes atrial disease not merely as a consequence of ventricular pathology or arrhythmia, but as a substrate with its own structural, functional, and thrombo-inflammatory implications.

We hope this collection will be both interesting and thought-provoking, offering readers concise, focused perspectives that encourage further discussion, research, and clinical attention to these important and sometimes underappreciated facets of cardiomyopathy.

Prim. Aleksandar Kibel, M.D., Ph.D.
Associate Professor,
Internal Medicine Specialist,
Cardiology Subspecialist,
International Medical Center Priora,
Head of Internal Medicine and Cardiology,
Head of the Scientific Unit for Medical Research,

Faculty of Medicine,
Department of Physiology and Immunology,
University of Osijek,
Osijek, Croatia

Faculty of Dental Medicine and Health,
Department of Clinical Medicine
University of Osijek,
Osijek, Croatia

Head of MEFOS2 Research Group of the Scientific Centre of Excellence
for Personalized Health Care,
University of Osijek,
Osijek, Croatia

Chapter 1

Immune Mechanisms in the Pathogenesis of Primary Cardiomyopathies

Dora Uršić and Aleksandar Kibel

Abstract

Among the many pathophysiological mechanisms that contribute to the occurrence, development and clinical course of cardiomyopathies, immune mechanisms play one of the important roles. While there is much more to be investigated, our understanding of underlying immune mechanisms has significantly improved over time, and we are starting to piece together a complex network of interactions that lead to the clinical manifestations of cardiomyopathies. This chapter aims to give a concise overview of some of the most important immune-mediated processes that are associated with the pathogenesis of primary cardiomyopathies, including hyperthrophic cardiomyopathy, arrhythmogenic cardiomyopathy, dilated cardiomyopathy, restrictive cardiomyopathy, but also of other types.

Keywords: immune system, inflammation, signaling pathways, hyperthrophic cardiomyopathy, arrhythmogenic cardiomyopathy, dilated cardiomyopathy, restrictive cardiomyopathy

1. Introduction

Our understanding regarding the development of cardiomyopathy (CMP) has improved over the last decades. Evolution of a cardiomyopathic presentation is determined by interplay between cellular signaling pathways, external influences and genetic profile [1]. Immune-mediated processes are fundamental to the pathogenesis and clinical evolution of diverse cardiomyopathy subtypes. Inflammatory mediators have been found to be elevated in both patients with acute decompensated heart failure and those with preserved ejection fraction [2, 3]. According to the "cytokine hypothesis," cytokine signaling pathways in the heart and bloodstream have an important role in the development of heart failure [4, 5]. In order to eradicate the pathogenic stimuli, inflammation serves as a physiological defense mechanism against various injuries. The inappropriate inflammatory response results in chronic inflammation and myocardial fibrosis. The heart responds to tissue damage by triggering both innate (macrophages, neutrophils, dendritic cells) and adaptive (T and B cells) immune responses (**Figure 1**) [6]. Progressive fibrosis results in dysfunction, scarring and myocardial injury [7]. Therefore, CMP patients may

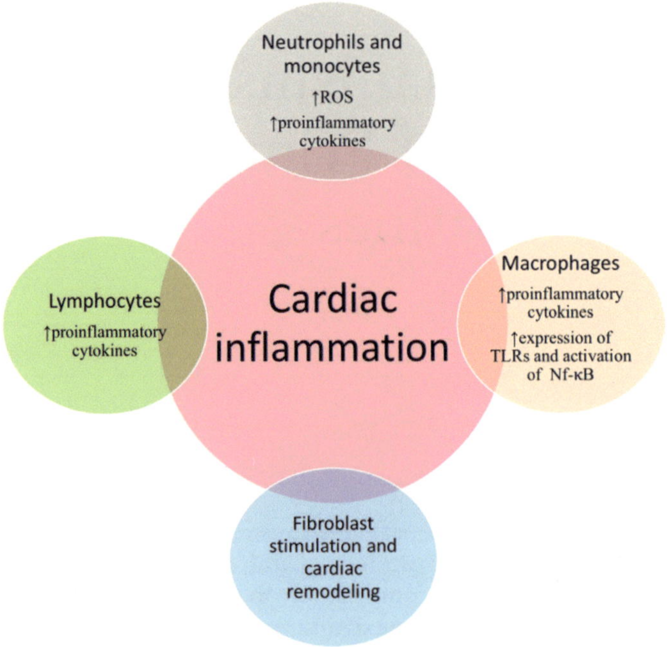

Figure 1.
Schematic overview of the cardiac inflammation.

exhibit a range of clinical presentations, from being asymptomatic to experiencing severe symptoms such as malignant arrhythmias, heart failure or sudden cardiac death [1]. Elucidating the immune mechanisms underlying CMPs is essential for developing novel diagnostic tools and therapies aimed at preventing or reversing adverse cardiac remodeling. Although immune-directed therapeutic approaches are actively pursued, the translation from experimental success to clinical efficacy remains challenging. The aim of this chapter is to provide an overview of key immune-mediated processes implicated in the pathogenesis of primary CMPs, including hypertrophic cardiomyopathy, arrhythmogenic cardiomyopathy, dilated cardiomyopathy, myocarditis, inflammatory cardiomyopathy, restrictive cardiomyopathy, stress-induced cardiomyopathy, tachycardia-induced cardiomyopathy and peripartum cardiomyopathy.

2. Hypertrophic cardiomyopathy

Hypertrophic cardiomyopathy (HCM) is a multifaced, autosomal dominant cardiovascular disease that often correlates with genetic mutations within genes that encode cardiac sarcomere proteins [8]. HCM manifests as fibrosis, reduced diastolic function and asymmetric thickening of the left ventricle (LV) [9]. The primary defect in the pathogenesis of HCM is gene mutation, which is directly responsible for altered transcription rate, translation efficiency and modifications in the structure and function of the sarcomeric proteins involved [1]. Advances in genetics have revealed more than 1000 mutations associated with HCM most frequently occurring in sarcomeric genes including β-cardiac myosin (MYH7) and cardiac myosin-binding protein-C (MYBPC3) [10]. The initial defect causes molecular changes, including the activation of calcium-sensitive and stress-responsive molecular pathways that induce myocardial hypertrophy and fibrosis [1]. However, data from clinical analysis and contemporary genetic studies indicate that single gene variants alone cannot fully account for the wide clinical variability seen in HCM. Recent utilization of network-based approaches in HCM research has uncovered a diverse array of protein-protein interactions that contribute to the disease's pathobiology, outside of the traditional contractile sarcomeric myofilaments [8].

Multiple studies have reported myocardial leukocyte infiltration and elevated inflammatory cytokines in patients with hypertrophic cardiomyopathy (HCM), including tumor necrosis factor-alpha (TNF-α), interleukin-6 (IL-6), as well as increased plasma concentrations of soluble Fas (sFas) and soluble Fas ligand (sFas-L) [11, 12]. Upon strong stimulation, leukocytes release nuclear contents such as neutrophil extracellular traps (NETs); these structures physically trap cells, fibrinogen and various proteins involved in inflammation, platelet aggregation and endothelial injury [13]. The pathogenesis of hypertrophic cardiomyopathy (HCM) progresses through several stages: an initial genetic predisposition characterized by sarcomeric gene mutations in approximately 40–60% of patients; an early stage marked by tissue inflammation and the formation of neutrophil extracellular traps (NETs); an intermediate phase involving platelet activation, microvascular thrombosis and transforming growth factor β1 (TGF-β1) signaling; and a late stage distinguished by myocardial fibrosis, ventricular disarray and hypertrophy (**Figure 2**) [1].

Recent studies suggest that necroptosis may be a key mechanism in HCM, with immune cell infiltration contributing to disease pathology. The predominant immune cells identified in myocardial tissue of HCM patients include monocytes, resting mast cells, regulatory T cells (Tregs), activated and resting natural killer (NK) cells, M2 macrophages, resting memory CD4+ T cells, naive B cells and eosinophils. Compared with controls, HCM patients show a marked decrease in M2 macrophages and resting dendritic cells, alongside the increased levels of monocytes and M0 macrophages [14]. Cardiac M2 macrophages are critical for maintaining cardiac homeostasis and play a vital role in tissue repair and regeneration following cardiac injury [15].

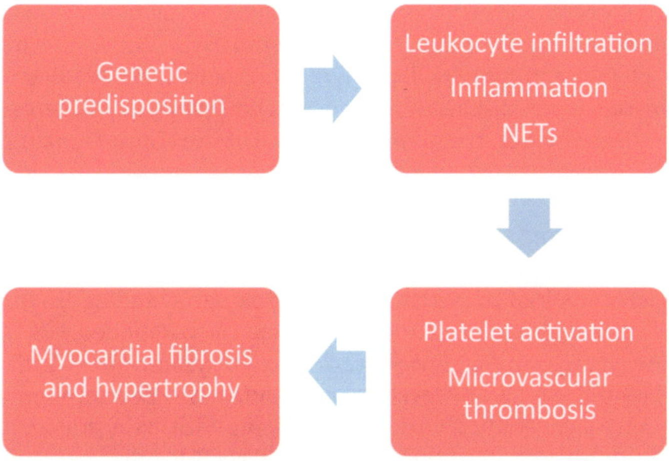

Figure 2.
Schematic overview of the hypertrophic cardiomyopathy (HCM) pathogenesis.

Bioinformatics analyses have revealed differential gene expression related to necroptosis between HCM tissues and normal myocardium. JAK2, BCL2 and CYBB have emerged as promising diagnostic biomarkers for HCM. CYBB expression positively correlates with M2 macrophages, whereas BCL2 and JAK2 show negative correlations [14]. JAK2, a member of the Janus kinase family, is highly expressed in HCM, with numerous studies demonstrating that its inhibition effectively suppresses apoptosis and associated signaling pathways. Dysregulation of the JAK2-STAT3 pathway has also been implicated in HCM pathogenesis. The increased activity of JAK2 in HCM may result from elevated IL-6 bioactivity and oxidative stress, which stimulate JAK2 signaling pathways involved in cardiac hypertrophy [16, 17]. BCL2, a regulatory member of the BCL protein family, plays a dual role in apoptosis regulation, exhibiting both proapoptotic and antiapoptotic functions [18]. It significantly contributes to the development of cardiac hypertrophy [19]. Pharmacological inhibitors targeting BCL2, including LY294002—an inhibitor of the PI3K/AKT signaling pathway—and Venetoclax, a selective BCL2 inhibitor, have demonstrated protective effects against cardiac hypertrophy by suppressing BCL2 activity [20]. The CYBB gene is responsible for the production of reactive oxygen species (ROS) in response to cytokine signaling. Upregulation of CYBB has been suggested as a potential biomarker for hypertrophic cardiomyopathy (HCM) [14]. Additionally, hearts affected by HCM exhibit global energetic impairment, demonstrated by reduced levels of high-energy phosphate metabolites such as ATP, ADP and phosphocreatine (PCr), along with decreased expression of mitochondrial genes involved in creatine kinase function and ATP generation. These mitochondrial defects are associated with increased ROS production and compromised antioxidant defenses [21].

3. Arrhythmogenic cardiomyopathy

Arrhythmogenic cardiomyopathy (ACM) is a myocardial disease characterized by progressive fibro-fatty replacement of the myocardium in the right and/or left ventricles, leading to gradual heart failure [22]. Dominant-right arrhythmogenic cardiomyopathy (ARVC) results from autosomal dominant mutations in genes encoding desmosomal proteins, including plakophilin-2 (PKP2), desmoplakin (DSP), plakoglobin (JUP), desmocollin-2 (DSC2), and desmoglein-2 (DSG2) [23]. Plakoglobin regulates transcription by competing with β-catenin in the Wnt/β-catenin signaling pathway through interactions with T cell/lymphoid-enhancing binding transcription factors [24]. Disruption of desmosomes and adherens junctions elevates mechanical stress on cardiomyocytes, triggering activation of the Hippo signaling pathway [25]. In contrast, dominant-left arrhythmogenic cardiomyopathy (ALVC) is linked to variants in non-desmosomal genes associated with arrhythmia, such as lamin A/C, phospholamban, and filamin-C [26]. Patchy infiltration of inflammatory cells is frequently observed in myocardial biopsies from ACM patients [2]. Compared to controls, plasma levels of proinflammatory cytokines including IL-1β, IL-6 and TNF-α, chemokines such as CCL-2 and CCL-3, and the components of the complement system are elevated in ACM patients, reflecting systemic para-inflammation [27, 28]. Autoimmunity is also believed to contribute to the development of ACM [29]. A recent flow cytometry study revealed that patients with arrhythmogenic cardiomyopathy (ACM) exhibit decreased frequencies of CD4+ T helper type 1 cells, natural killer (NK) cells and terminally differentiated CD8+ EMRA+ T cells compared to

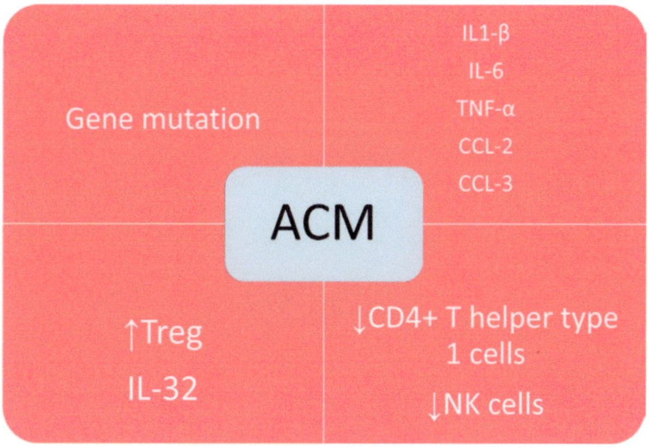

Figure 3.
Schematic overview of the arrhythmogenic cardiomyopathy (ACM) pathogenesis.

age-matched healthy controls. Conversely, an increased proportion of effector/memory FOXP3+ CCR4+ CD45RO+ regulatory CD4+ T cells (Tregs) was observed in ACM patients. Interleukin 32 (IL-32) emerged as the most differentially expressed gene in Tregs from ACM patients relative to controls. IL-32 is implicated in promoting cardiac remodeling and dysfunction in ACM through mechanisms involving lipid deposition and collagen accumulation. Regulatory T cells are crucial for maintaining immune tolerance and modulating inflammation; however, in ACM, the interplay between autoimmune reactions and genetically driven myocardial injury may provoke exaggerated immune activation that Tregs attempt to mitigate. Elevated IL-32 expression by Tregs in ACM may contribute to pathologic cardiac remodeling, suggesting IL-32 as the promising therapeutic target to counteract fibrofatty myocardial remodeling characteristic of the disease (**Figure 3**) [30].

4 Dilated cardiomyopathy

Dilated cardiomyopathy (DCM) is a condition defined by left ventricular enlargement and impaired systolic function, excluding secondary causes such as hypertension, valvular, congenital, or ischemic heart disease [31]. Genetic mutations are responsible for approximately 35% of DCM cases, while the remaining cases are attributed to various environmental factors such as infectious, toxic, and metabolic causes of myocardial dysfunction [31, 32].

Dilated inflammatory cardiomyopathy (DCMi) describes a group of disorders characterized by heart muscle inflammation leading to a dilated heart and impaired myocardial function. Globally, infectious myocarditis is the primary cause of DCMi [33].

Myocardial injury induces stimulation of the innate and adaptive immune systems. These immune cells and their secreted cytokines can amplify inflammatory and autoimmune responses, leading to fibrosis and structural remodeling of the heart tissue (**Figure 4**) [1].

Elevated cytokine levels promote the mobilization of neutrophils and monocytes into the myocardium, thereby intensifying inflammation. Activated NOD-like

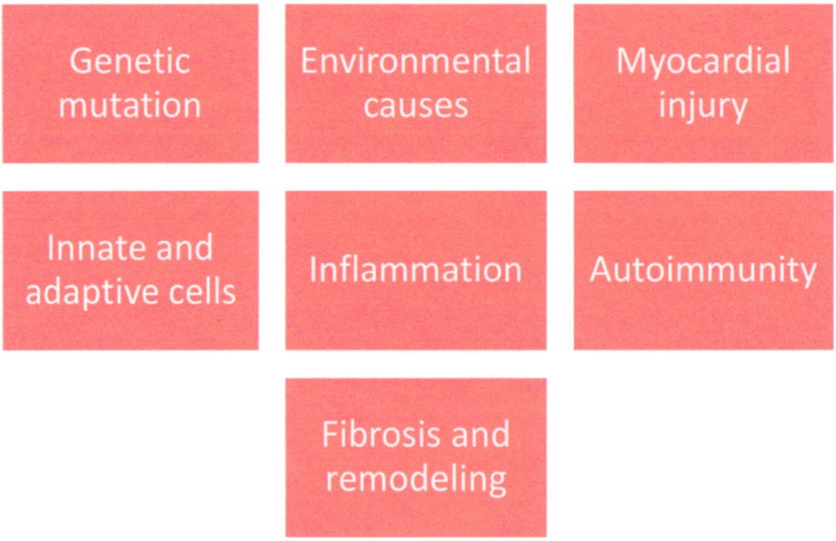

Figure 4.
Schematic overview of the dilated cardiomyopathy (DCM) pathogenesis.

receptor protein 3 (NLRP3) inflammasome in neutrophils can induce chronic inflammation during DCM development *via* Sirtuin 2 (SIRT2)-dependent manner. Additionally, increased levels of myeloid differentiation factor-2 (MD-2) in DCM patients enhance the pro-inflammatory activity of monocytes, leading to elevated cytokine production and stimulation of endothelial cell-mediated monocyte recruitment *via* the TLR4/NF-κB signaling pathway [34]. Recruited monocytes can differentiate into tissue-resident macrophages. Different origins of macrophages can either promote or mitigate DCM by modulating the expression of specific immune molecules and influencing the migration and accumulation of inflammatory cells. In the myocardial tissue, recruited monocytes differentiate into CCR2- (C-C chemokine receptor 2) and CCR2 + macrophages. CCR2-macrophages enhance the production of pro-angiogenic growth factors and facilitate adaptive remodeling of the heart. On the other hand, CCR2 + macrophages may facilitate monocyte mobilization through a myeloid differentiation primary response 88 (MYD88)-dependent mechanism in mouse models, leading to the secretion of monocyte chemoattractant proteins (MCPs) and subsequent monocyte migration [35, 36].

A decrease in invariant natural killer T (iNKT) cells in DCM contributes to increased myocardial fibrosis and impaired vasculogenesis, mediated by interferon-gamma (IFN-γ) [34, 37]. Dendritic cells can induce TCD4 + T cell activation in the myocardium and DCM when stimulated by toll-like receptors (TLRs) [38]. Several triggers activate adaptive immune cells and produce numerous cytokines and anti-heart autoantibodies (AHAs), promoting/inhibiting immune-inflammatory, fibrosis and remodeling in DCM [34].

In patients with *idiopathic dilated cardiomyopathy (iDCM)*, there is a notable activation of CD4+ T cells in the peripheral blood. This condition is marked by an imbalance between Th1 and Th2 cell populations, with an increase in Th1 cells and a decrease in Th2 cells. This imbalance may be associated with polymorphisms in the gene encoding cytotoxic T lymphocyte-associated antigen-4 (CTLA-4). Th1 cells present in the blood and myocardium contribute significantly to the development of DCM by secreting cytokines like IFN-γ, IL-2 and IL-12. The cytokines IL-2 and IL-12 stimulate the expansion of myocardial myosin-specific Th1 cells, which escalates autoimmune damage to the heart, while IFN-γ activates macrophages and mediates cytotoxic effects that help limit the progression of the disease [39, 40].

The differentiation of CD4+ T cells into Th17 cells is a crucial step in progression of autoimmune-related DCM and acute viral myocarditis. Studies indicates that Th17 cells are active during the acute phase aligned with viral presence, while Th2 cells become more prominent in the chronic phase of DCM [34, 41]. Regulatory T cells (Tregs) are fundamental for maintaining autoimmune tolerance. A recent bioinformatics study suggested that the upregulation of follicular helper T cells (Tfh) driven by CD48 and CD3D may be one of the immunological mechanisms associated with the onset of DCM [42].

B cells contribute to autoimmunity in DCM by producing AHAs through molecular mimicry triggered by viral exposure. Moreover, B cells release a range of pro-inflammatory and anti-inflammatory cytokines that participate in the immunoinflammatory processes underlying DCM [43]. TNF-α-secreting B cells were reportedly significantly increased in DCM patients with a history of viral myocarditis. TNF-α contributes to the promotion of myocardial fibrosis and inflammation by modulating the secretory profile of myocardial fibroblasts and activating the ERK1/2 signaling pathway [44, 45]. Secretion of natural IgM was also found to be decreased in iDCM patients [46]. Specific immune cells and their associated cytokines are essential in the immunopathogenesis of DCM and represent the promising targets for therapeutic intervention. Rituximab, an anti-CD20 monoclonal antibody, has demonstrated positive outcomes in 53% of patients with DCMi associated with CD20+ B-lymphocytes [47]. In addition, inhibition of IL-1 has the potential to enhance cardiac function and reduce myocardial inflammation in DCMi [48]. Immunoadsorption effectively removes anti-heart autoantibodies (AHAs) from plasma, leading to improved hemodynamic function [49]. Intravenous immunoglobulin (IVIG) therapy has been shown to suppress inflammatory cytokines, regulate T and B cell activity and improve cardiac function; however, these functional improvements are not observed in patients with advanced disease stages [34].

5. Myocarditis and inflammatory cardiomyopathy

Myocarditis is a condition characterized by inflammation of the heart muscle, confirmed through recognized histological, immunological and immunohistochemical diagnostic criteria [50]. When myocardial dysfunction is present alongside biopsy-confirmed myocarditis, the condition is referred to as inflammatory cardiomyopathy. Autoimmunity plays an important role in myocarditis, occurring either as myocardial damage following an infection or as a primary autoimmune disease targeting the heart [51]. HLA-DR4, HLA-DR12 and HLA-DR15 alleles have been linked with the onset of myocarditis and an elevated risk of progression to DCM. Recent research has identified a greater frequency of HLA-DQ1 presence in individuals diagnosed with myocarditis in contrast to individuals without the condition [52]. Myocarditis results from a complex interaction involving various pro-inflammatory cells, including monocytes CX3CR1+, CCR2+ macrophages, dendritic cells, eosinophils, Th1, Th2, Th17 and Treg (**Table 1**) [53].

Cells/cytokines	Role
CCR2+ macrophages	Recruited to the heart from peripheral CD11b + monocytes
	Pro-inflammatory
Granulocytes	Pro-inflammatory cells recruitment
Eosinophils	Secretion of Il-4, IL-5
Dendritic cells	Accumulation in the myocardium
	Induction of Th1 and Th17 differentiation
Th17	Secretion of Il-17
	Th17/reg ratio in favor of Th17
Th1	Recruitment of CD8 + Ly
Th2	Secretion of IL-4
	Dual role
IL-1β, IL-4, IL-6, IL-17, IL-22, IL-23, TNF-α, TGF-β1	Pro-inflammatory
	Myocarditis development
IL-10	Anti-inflammatory
	Reduced in myocarditis

Table 1.
The role of cellular immunity and cytokines in the pathogenesis of myocarditis.

6. Restrictive cardiomyopathy

Restrictive cardiomyopathy (RCM) is a heart muscle condition caused by increased stiffness of the myocardium, resulting in compromised ventricular filling [54]. RCM can be idiopathic, hereditary or secondary to systemic conditions like amyloidosis, sarcoidosis and hereditary hemochromatosis. About 30% of RCM cases have a familial background, regarded as a primary genetic disease. Nevertheless, only a limited number of genes—including those encoding cardiac troponin T (cTnT), troponin I (cTnI), myosin-binding protein C (MYBPC), MYH7, myosin light chains 2 and 3 (MYL2, MYL3), desmin (DES), MYPN, titin (TTN), Bcl2-associated athanogene 3 (BAG3), discoidin, CUB and LCCL domain-containing 2 (DCBLD2), lamin A/C (LMNA) and filamin C (FLNC) have been linked to familial RCM. Genetic mutations linked to inherited RCM mainly affect the structural proteins of the sarcomere [55].

6.1 Cardiac amyloidosis

Cardiac amyloidosis results from the accumulation of amyloid proteins within the extracellular space of the heart muscle [56]. The two primary forms are AL amyloidosis, which is derived from immunoglobulin light chains, and ATTR amyloidosis, which originates from transthyretin protein. These represent the predominant types of amyloidosis found in patients with cardiac involvement. Patients with this condition experience cardiac inflammation marked by increased levels of CD3-positive T cells, CD68-positive macrophages and elevated pro-inflammatory cytokines including TNF-α, IL-1β, IL-6 and IL-10 (**Figure 5**) [57, 58]. In recent study, myocardial

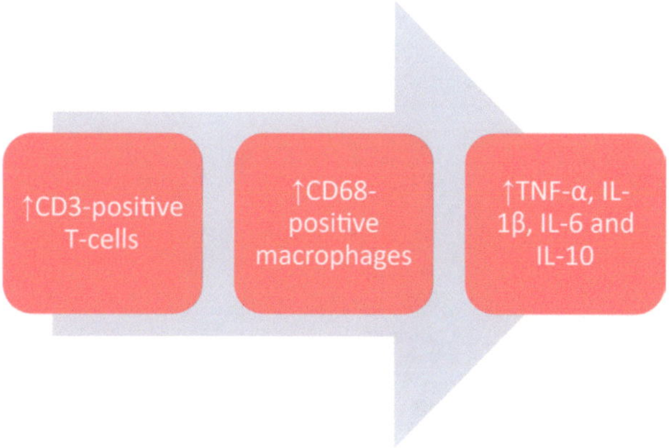

Figure 5.
Schematic overview of the cardiac amyloidosis pathogenesis.

tissue samples from 157 patients with cardiac amyloidosis (46.5% AL type, 53.3% ATTR type) were examined using immunohistochemistry to evaluate the presence and quantity of T lymphocytes (CD3), macrophages (CD68) and neutrophils (MPO). A strong association has been observed between the quantity of macrophages present in the myocardium and the New York Heart Association (NYHA) functional class [59].

6.2 Cardiac sarcoidosis

Cardiac sarcoidosis (CS) is a multi-system inflammatory disorder of unknown etiology characterized by the formation of non-caseating granulomas [60]. Studies have shown an association between HLA class II alleles and the risk of developing sarcoidosis and the severity of disease [61, 62]. The T-cell immune response is disrupted, marked by the activation of Th1 cells that secrete cytokines such as IFN-γ, TNF-α, TGF-β, IL-2 and IL-12 [63]. This is followed by an anti-inflammatory Th2 type immune response characterized by the presence of cytokines such as IL-4, IL-5, IL-10 and IL-13 [64]. The regulatory T-cell response is impaired, resulting in persistent local effector T-cell response to tissue antigens. The immune system dysregulation ultimately leads to activation of macrophages and formation of noncaseating granulomas. An active inflammatory phase may develop into a fibrotic phase, with both stages potentially contributing to impaired cardiac function (**Figure 6**) [65, 66].

The fibrotic remodeling of chronic granulomas occurs through a shift toward a Th2-type immune response, which involves molecules such as platelet-derived growth factor-B (PDGF-B), insulin-like growth factor 1 (IGF-1) and insulin-like growth factor binding protein-related protein 2 (IGFBP-2) [64].

6.3 Anderson–Fabry disease

Anderson–Fabry disease (AFD) is the most prevalent storage disorder and an occasional cause of RCM. It is an X-linked recessive condition caused by mutations in the GLA gene, leading to deficient or absent α-galactosidase A (GLA) enzyme activity, which results in the gradual buildup of globotriaosylceramide (Gb3) in various tissues. The typical manifestation of cardiac involvement in AFD is cardiac hypertrophy,

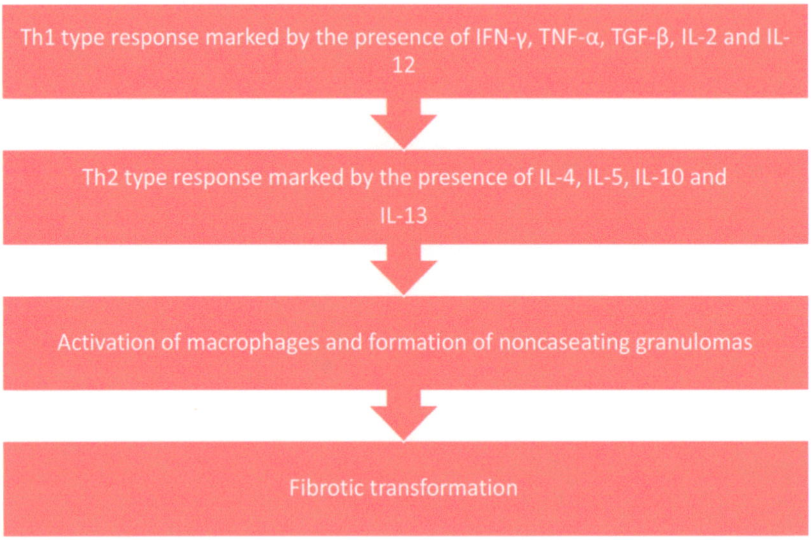

Figure 6.
Schematic overview of the cardiac sarcoidosis (CS) pathogenesis.

which may worsen and lead to impaired contractility and diastolic filling [67]. Some studies reported that accumulation of Gb3 induces progressive lysosomal and cellular dysfunction, which subsequently triggers signaling pathways that result in hypertrophy, necrosis and fibrosis. Organ damage in AFD cannot be solely attributed to the mechanical accumulation of glycosphingolipids. Lysosomal storage materials also contribute by causing mitochondrial dysfunction. This dysfunction is characterized by reduced activity of respiratory chain enzymes and a consequent depletion of energy-rich phosphate compounds, which are crucial for cellular energy metabolism [68]. Inflammation could play a pivotal role in the onset and progression of cardiac alterations seen in AFD, contributing significantly to the disease's cardiac pathology (**Figure** 7).

In end-stage cardiomyopathy in patients with AFD, fibrosis in the left ventricle is a common finding [69]. A study investigating cardiomyocyte dysfunction in patients AFD and cardiomyopathy found that the accumulation of GB3 within cells is associated with oxidative damage to proteins and DNA, leading to impaired cardiomyocyte

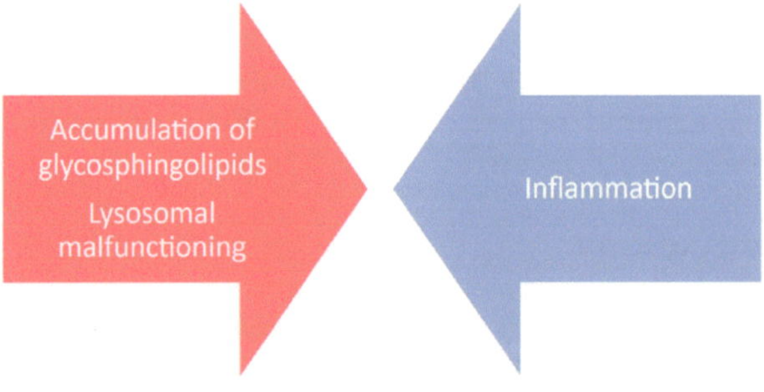

Figure 7.
Schematic overview of the Anderson–Fabry disease (AFD) pathogenesis.

function and cell death. Study also showed that several cytokines' levels (IL-1β, TNF-α, IL-6, monocyte chemoattractant protein-1 (MCP-1), intercellular adhesion molecule-1 and soluble vascular adhesion molecule) were increased in the serum of AFD patients. These findings suggest that proinflammatory cytokines play a crucial role in promoting the advancement of cardiomyopathy associated with AFD [70].

7. Stress-induced cardiomyopathy

Takotsubo syndrome (TTS) or stress-induced cardiomyopathy is an acute heart failure condition marked by temporary ventricular dysfunction and diverse abnormalities of the ventricular wall caused by excessive sympathetic nervous system activation [71]. TTS involves a pronounced acute inflammatory reaction driven mainly by innate immune cells, which gradually subsides into a chronic inflammation. Overstimulation of cardiac β-adrenoreceptors in mice triggers activation of the NLRP3 inflammasome, leading to elevated secretion of the IL-18, but not IL-1β [72]. This leads to cardiac inflammation driven by galectin-3, accompanied by macrophage infiltration, which subsequently causes pathological remodeling and impaired cardiac function [73]. Increased levels of IL-6 and IL-10 were observed acutely in TTS [74]. Studies of patient endomyocardial biopsies have shown macrophage infiltration in TTS hearts [75, 76]. Furthermore, histological staining revealed that neutrophils, along with CD3+ T cells and CD20+ B cells, are the components of the acute myocardial inflammatory infiltrate in TTS [75]. During the acute phase of TTS, an increase in classical CD14++CD16− monocytes and a decrease in intermediate CD14++CD16+ plus non-classical CD14 + CD16++ monocytes were observed in patients' blood. Following myocardial injury in TTS, classical monocytes may enter the heart tissue, where they contribute to inflammation and subsequently differentiate into macrophages [77].

7.1 Peripartum cardiomyopathy

Tachycardiomyopathy or tachycardia-induced cardiomyopathy (TCM) has long been recognized as a reversible form of nonischemic cardiomyopathy. TCM features alterations in cardiomyocyte structure and mitochondrial arrangement, alongside cardiac inflammation largely driven by macrophages. In contrast to patients with DCM, patients with TCM exhibited increased myocardial expression of major histocompatibility complex class II molecules along with a higher infiltration of CD68+ macrophages. Myocardial fibrosis occurs to a significantly lesser extent in TCM patients compared to those with DCM. Additionally, a disturbed distribution pattern of mitochondria was predominantly present in TCM [78].

Peripartum cardiomyopathy (PPCM) is an uncommon form of heart failure that arises during the final month of pregnancy or within several months following childbirth, occurring without any other identifiable cause of heart failure [79]. Multiple factors may contribute to PPCM, such as the hemodynamic stress of pregnancy, vascular and hormonal influences, inflammation, immune responses and genetic predispositions [80]. It has been shown that the absence of cardiac peroxisome proliferator-activated receptor-gamma coactivator-1 alpha (PGC-1α) in mice results in the onset of PPCM. The human placenta produces soluble fms-like tyrosine kinase 1 (sFlt-1) during the later stages of pregnancy. The antiangiogenic environment created by sFlt-1 is linked to cardiac dysfunction, as evidenced by unusually high serum sFlt-1 levels found in women with PPCM [80, 81]. Removing STAT3 specifically from cardiomyocytes in mice results in the onset of PPCM. Also, patients with PPCM exhibit the elevated levels of the 16-kDa prolactin fragment alongside decreased STAT3 levels [82]. Plasma levels of microRNA 146a (miR-146a) and Fas/APO-1 were found to be elevated in women with PPCM, promoting the apoptosis of cardiomyocytes [83]. The TTN gene, which encodes the sarcomere protein titin, as well as FLNC, DSP and BAG3, have been linked with PPCM [84]. β1-Adrenergic receptor autoantibodies (β1R-AAs) and M2-muscarinic receptor autoantibodies (M2R-AABs) could be participating in PPCM pathogenesis [85].

8. Conclusion

Immune-mediated processes, including chronic inflammation, autoimmunity and dysregulated immune responses, fundamentally drive myocardial remodeling, fibrosis and functional impairment in CMPs. The immunopathogenesis of primary CMPs remains only partially understood, despite continuous advancement in both experimental models and clinical research. Anti-inflammatory strategies targeting inflammatory modulation constitute a promising therapeutic approach for CMPs; however, further studies are essential to elucidate immunologic mechanisms and discover the additional molecular targets.

Author details

Dora Uršić[1,2] and Aleksandar Kibel[3,4,5]*

1 Department of Rheumatology, Clinical Immunology and Allergology, University Hospital Center Osijek, Osijek, Croatia

2 Faculty of Medicine Osijek, Josip Juraj Strossmayer University of Osijek, Osijek, Croatia

3 Scientific Unit for Medical Research, International Medical Center Prioran, Cepi, Croatia

4 Department of Physiology and Immunology, Faculty of Medicine Osijek, Josip Juraj Strossmayer University of Osijek, Osijek, Croatia

5 Department of Clinical Medicine Faculty of Dental Medicine and Health, Josip Juraj Strossmayer University of Osijek, Osijek, Croatia

*Address all correspondence to: aleksandar_mf@yahoo.com; aleksandar.kibel@priora.eu; aleksandar.kibel@mefos.hr

References

[1] Monda E, Palmiero G, Rubino M, et al. Molecular basis of inflammation in the pathogenesis of cardiomyopathies. International Journal of Molecular Sciences. 2020;**21**(18):6462

[2] Thiene G, Corrado D, Nava A, et al. Right ventricular cardiomyopathy: Is there evidence of an inflammatory aetiology? European Heart Journal. 1991;**12**(Suppl. D):22-25

[3] Matsumori A, Yamada T, Suzuki H, Matoba Y, Sasayama S. Increased circulating cytokines in patients with myocarditis and cardiomyopathy. British Heart Journal. 1994;**72**(6):561-566

[4] Seta Y, Shan K, Bozkurt B, Oral H, Mann DL. Basic mechanisms in heart failure: The cytokine hypothesis. Journal of Cardiac Failure. 1996;**2**:243-249

[5] Mann DL. Innate immunity and the failing heart: The cytokine hypothesis revisited. Circulation Research. 2015;**116**(7):1254-1268

[6] Lee SB, Kalluri R. Mechanistic connection between inflammation and fibrosis. Kidney International. Supplement. 2010;**119**:S22-S26

[7] Coggins M, Rosenzweig A. The fire within: Cardiac inflammatory signaling in health and disease. Circulation Research. 2012;**110**(1):116-125

[8] Maron BA, Wang RS, Carnethon MR, et al. What causes hypertrophic cardiomyopathy? The American Journal of Cardiology. 2022;**179**:74-82

[9] Marian AJ, Braunwald E. Hypertrophic cardiomyopathy: Genetics, pathogenesis, clinical manifestations, diagnosis, and therapy. Circulation Research. 2017;**121**:749-770

[10] Spudich JA. Three perspectives on the molecular basis of hypercontractility caused by hypertrophic cardiomyopathy mutations. Pflügers Archiv. 2019;**471**:701-717

[11] Zen K, Irie H, Doue T, et al. Analysis of circulating apoptosis mediators and proinflammatory cytokines in patients with idiopathic hypertrophic cardiomyopathy: Comparison between nonobstructive and dilated-phase hypertrophic cardiomyopathy. International Heart Journal. 2005;**46**:231-244

[12] Högye M, Mándi Y, Csanády M, et al. Comparison of circulating levels of interleukin-6 and tumor necrosis factor-alpha in hypertrophic cardiomyopathy and in idiopathic dilated cardiomyopathy. The American Journal of Cardiology. 2004;**94**:249-251

[13] Becker RC, Owens AP III, Sadayappan S. Tissue-level inflammation and ventricular remodeling in hypertrophic cardiomyopathy. Journal of Thrombosis and Thrombolysis. 2020;**49**:177-183

[14] Hou C, Fei S, Jia F. Necroptosis and immune infiltration in hypertrophic cardiomyopathy: Novel insights from bioinformatics analyses. Frontiers in Cardiovascular Medicine. 2024;**11**:1293786

[15] Moskalik A, Niderla-Bielińska J, Ratajska A. Multiple roles of cardiac macrophages in heart homeostasis and failure. Heart Failure Reviews. 2022;**27**(4):1413-1430

[16] Maron BA, Wang RS, Shevtsov S, et al. Individualized interactomes for network-based precision medicine in hypertrophic cardiomyopathy with implications for other clinical pathophenotypes. Nature Communications. 2021;**12**(1):873

[17] Marian AJ, Senthil V, Chen SN, et al. Antifibrotic effects of antioxidant N-acetylcysteine in a mouse model of human hypertrophic cardiomyopathy mutation. Journal of the American College of Cardiology. 2006;**47**(4):827-834

[18] Czabotar PE, Lessene G, Strasser A, Adams JM. Control of apoptosis by the BCL-2 protein family: Implications for physiology and therapy. Nature Reviews. Molecular Cell Biology. 2014;**15**(1):49-63

[19] Buzás K, Megyeri K, Hõgye M, et al. Comparative study of the roles of cytokines and apoptosis in dilated and hypertrophic cardiomyopathies. European Cytokine Network. 2004;**15**(1):53-59

[20] Meng X, Cui J, He G. Bcl-2 is involved in cardiac hypertrophy through PI3K-akt pathway. BioMed Research International. 2021;**2021**:6615502

[21] Ranjbarvaziri S, Kooiker KB, Ellenberger M, et al. Altered cardiac energetics and mitochondrial dysfunction in hypertrophic cardiomyopathy. Circulation. 2021;**144**(21):1714-1731

[22] Chen S, Chen L, Duru F, Hu S. Heart failure in patients with arrhythmogenic cardiomyopathy. Journal of Clinical Medicine. 2021;**10**:4782

[23] Huynh K. Increased degradation of desmosomal proteins in ACM. Nature Reviews. Cardiology. 2023;**20**:371

[24] Zhurinsky J, Shtutman M, Ben-Ze'Ev A. Plakoglobin and beta-catenin: Protein interactions, regulation and biological roles. Journal of Cell Science. 2000;**113**:3127-3139

[25] Hu Y, Pu WT. Hippo activation in arrhythmogenic cardiomyopathy. Circulation Research. 2014;**114**:402-405

[26] Kumar S, Baldinger SH, Gandjbakhch E, et al. Long-term arrhythmic and nonarrhythmic outcomes of Lamin A/C mutation carriers. Journal of the American College of Cardiology. 2016;**68**:2299-2307

[27] Campian ME, Verberne HJ, Hardziyenka M, et al. Assessment of inflammation in patients with arrhythmogenic right ventricular cardiomyopathy/dysplasia. European Journal of Nuclear Medicine and Molecular Imaging. 2010;**37**:2079-2085

[28] Ren J, Chen L, Chen X, et al. Acylation-stimulating protein and heart failure progression in arrhythmogenic right ventricular cardiomyopathy. ESC Heart Failure. 2023;**10**:492-501

[29] Caforio ALP, Re F, Avella A, et al. Evidence from family studies for autoimmunity in arrhythmogenic right ventricular cardiomyopathy. Circulation. 2020;**141**:1238-1248

[30] Soussi S, Maione AS, Lefèvre L, et al. Analysis of effector/memory regulatory T cells from arrhythmogenic cardiomyopathy patients identified IL-32 as a novel player in ACM pathogenesis. Cell Death & Disease. 2025;**16**(1):87

[31] Elliott PM, Andersson B, Arbustini E, et al. Classification of the cardiomyopathies: A position statement from the European Society of Cardiology Working Group on Myocardial and

pericardial diseases. European Heart Journal. 2008;**29**:270-276

[32] Pérez-Serra A, Toro R, Sarquella-Brugada G, et al. Genetic basis of dilated cardiomyopathy. International Journal of Cardiology. 2016;**224**:461-472

[33] Imanaka-Yoshida K. Inflammation in myocardial disease: From myocarditis to dilated cardiomyopathy. Pathology International. 2020;**70**:1-11

[34] Zhang J, Cheng L, Li Z, et al. Immune cells and related cytokines in dilated cardiomyopathy. Biomedicine & Pharmacotherapy. 2024;**171**:116159

[35] Chaffin M, Papangeli I, Simonson B, et al. Single-nucleus profiling of human dilated and hypertrophic cardiomyopathy. Nature. 2022;**608**(7921):174-180

[36] Bajpai G, Bredemeyer A, Li W, et al. Tissue resident CCR2- and CCR2+ cardiac macrophages differentially orchestrate monocyte recruitment and fate specification following myocardial injury. Circulation Research. 2019;**124**(2):263-278

[37] Ong S, Ligons DL, Barin JG, et al. Natural killer cells limit cardiac inflammation and fibrosis by halting eosinophil infiltration. The American Journal of Pathology. 2015;**185**(3):847-861

[38] Eriksson U, Ricci R, Hunziker L, et al. Dendritic cell-induced autoimmune heart failure requires cooperation between adaptive and innate immunity. Nature Medicine. 2003;**9**(12):1484-1490

[39] Liu W, Li WM, Gao C, et al. Relationship of CTLA-4 exon 1 A49-->G polymorphism with sCTLA-4 and Th1/Th2 bias in idiopathic dilated cardiomyopathy. Zhonghua Yi Xue Za Zhi. 2005;**85**(45):3221-3224

[40] Efthimiadis I, Skendros P, Sarantopoulos A, Boura P. CD4+/CD25+ T-lymphocytes and Th1/Th2 regulation in dilated cardiomyopathy. Hippokratia. 2011;**15**(4):335-342

[41] Yuan J, Cao AL, Yu M, et al. Th17 cells facilitate the humoral immune response in patients with acute viral myocarditis. Journal of Clinical Immunology. 2010;**30**(2):226-234

[42] Gan T, Hu J, Aledan AKO, et al. Exploring the pathogenesis and immune infiltration in dilated cardiomyopathy complicated with atrial fibrillation by bioinformatics analysis. Frontiers in Immunology. 2023;**14**:1049351

[43] Matsumoto Y, Park IK, Kohyama K. B-cell epitope spreading is a critical step for the switch from C-protein-induced myocarditis to dilated cardiomyopathy. The American Journal of Pathology. 2007;**170**(1):43-51

[44] Yu M, Wen S, Wang M, et al. TNF-α-secreting B cells contribute to myocardial fibrosis in dilated cardiomyopathy. Journal of Clinical Immunology. 2013;**33**(5):1002-1008

[45] Bräuninger H, Thottakara T, Schön J, et al. Cytokine-mediated alterations of human cardiac fibroblast's secretome. International Journal of Molecular Sciences. 2021;**22**(22):12262

[46] Tang Q, Cen Z, Lu J, et al. The abnormal distribution of peripheral B1 cells and transition B cells in patients with idiopathic dilated cardiomyopathy: A pilot study. BMC Cardiovascular Disorders. 2022;**22**(1):78

[47] Tschöpe C, Van Linthout S, Spillmann F, et al. Targeting CD20+ B-lymphocytes in inflammatory dilated cardiomyopathy with rituximab improves clinical course: A case series.

European Heart Journal - Case Reports. 2019;**3**(3):ytz131

[48] De Luca G, Campochiaro C, Dinarello CA, et al. Treatment of dilated cardiomyopathy with interleukin-1 inhibition. Annals of Internal Medicine. 2018;**169**(11):819-820

[49] Bian RT, Wang ZT, Li WY. Immunoadsorption treatment for dilated cardiomyopathy: A PRISMA-compliant systematic review and meta-analysis. Medicine (Baltimore). 2021;**100**(26):e26475

[50] Caforio AL, Pankuweit S, Arbustini E, et al. Current state of knowledge on aetiology, diagnosis, management, and therapy of myocarditis: A position statement of the European Society of Cardiology Working Group on myocardial and pericardial diseases. European Heart Journal. 2013;**34**(33):2636-2648

[51] Caforio AL, Calabrese F, Angelini A, et al. A prospective study of biopsy-proven myocarditis: Prognostic relevance of clinical and aetiopathogenetic features at diagnosis. European Heart Journal. 2007;**28**(11):132-633

[52] Martinetti M, Dugoujon JM, Caforio AL, et al. HLA and immunoglobulin polymorphisms in idiopathic dilated cardiomyopathy. Human Immunology. 1992;**35**(3): 193-199

[53] Vicenzetto C, Giordani AS, Menghi C, et al. Cellular immunology of myocarditis: Lights and shades—A literature review. Cells. 2024;**13**(24): 2082

[54] Dadson K, Hauck L, Billia F. Molecular mechanisms in cardiomyopathy. Clinical Science. 2017;**131**:1375-1392

[55] Chintanaphol M, Orgil BO, Alberson NR, et al. Restrictive cardiomyopathy: From genetics and clinical overview to animal modeling. Reviews in Cardiovascular Medicine. 2022;**23**(3):108

[56] Nijst P, Tang WW. Recent advances in the diagnosis and management of amyloid cardiomyopathy. Faculty Reviews. 2021;**10**:31

[57] Chirinos JA, Orlenko A, Zhao L, et al. Multiple plasma biomarkers for risk stratification in patients with heart failure and preserved ejection fraction. Journal of the American College of Cardiology. 2020;**75**(11):1281-1295

[58] Hahn VS, Yanek LR, Vaishnav J, et al. Endomyocardial biopsy characterization of heart failure with preserved ejection fraction and prevalence of cardiac amyloidosis. JACC: Heart Failure. 2020;**8**(9):712-724

[59] Simon P, Behrens HM, Kristen A, Röcken C. Myocardial inflammatory cells in cardiac amyloidosis. Scientific Reports. 2024;**14**(1):23313

[60] Trivieri MG, Spagnolo P, Birnie D, Liu P, et al. Challenges in cardiac and pulmonary sarcoidosis: JACC state-of-the-art review. Journal of the American College of Cardiology. 2020;**76**(16):1878-1901

[61] Moller DR, Rybicki BA, Hamzeh NY, et al. Genetic, immunologic, and environmental basis of sarcoidosis. Annals of the American Thoracic Society. 2017;**14**:S429-S436

[62] Grunewald J, Kaiser Y, Ostadkarampour M, et al. T-cell receptor-HLA-DRB1 associations suggest specific antigens in pulmonary sarcoidosis. The European Respiratory Journal. 2016;**47**:898-909

[63] Hamzeh N, Steckman DA, Sauer WH, et al. Pathophysiology and clinical management of cardiac sarcoidosis. Nature Reviews. Cardiology. 2015;**12**:278-288

[64] Lagana SM, Parwani AV, Nichols LC. Cardiac sarcoidosis: A pathology-focused review. Archives of Pathology & Laboratory Medicine. 2010;**134**(7):1039-1046

[65] Grunewald J, Grutters JC, Arkema EV, Saketkoo LA, Moller DR, Muller-Quernheim J. Sarcoidosis. Nature Reviews. Disease Primers. 2019;**5**:45

[66] Cheng RK, Kittleson MM, Beavers CJ, et al. American Heart Association heart failure and transplantation Committee of the Council on clinical cardiology, and council on cardiovascular and stroke nursing. Diagnosis and Management of Cardiac Sarcoidosis: A scientific statement from the American Heart Association. Circulation. 2024;**149**(21):e1197-e1216

[67] Tuttolomondo A, Simonetta I, Riolo R, et al. Pathogenesis and molecular mechanisms of Anderson–Fabry disease and possible new molecular addressed therapeutic strategies. Inte+rnational Journal of Molecular Sciences. 2021;**22**(18):10088

[68] Ashrafian H, Redwood C, Blair E, et al. Hypertrophic cardiomyopathy: A paradigm for myocardial energy depletion. Trends in Genetics. 2003;**19**(5):263-268

[69] Niemann M, Breunig F, Beer M, Herrmann S, et al. The right ventricle in Fabry disease: Natural history and impact of enzyme replacement therapy. Heart. 2010;**96**(23):1915-1919

[70] Chimenti C, Scopelliti F, Vulpis E, et al. Increased oxidative stress contributes to cardiomyocyte dysfunction and death in patients with Fabry disease cardiomyopathy. Human Pathology. 2015;**46**(11):1760-1768

[71] Ghadri JR, Wittstein IS, Prasad A, et al. International expert consensus document on Takotsubo syndrome (Part I): Clinical characteristics, diagnostic criteria, and pathophysiology. European Heart Journal. 2018;**39**: 2032-2046

[72] Xiao H, Li H, Wang JJ, Zhang JS, et al. IL-18 cleavage triggers cardiac inflammation and fibrosis upon β-adrenergic insult. European Heart Journal. 2018;**39**(1):60-69

[73] Hu G, Wu J, Gu H, et al. Galectin-3-centered paracrine network mediates cardiac inflammation and fibrosis upon β-adrenergic insult. Science China. Life Sciences. 2023;**66**(5):1067-1078

[74] Santoro F, Tarantino N, Ferraretti A, et al. Serum interleukin 6 and 10 levels in Takotsubo cardiomyopathy: Increased admission levels may predict adverse events at follow-up. Atherosclerosis. 2016;**254**:28-34

[75] Wilson HM, Cheyne L, Brown P, et al. Characterization of the myocardial inflammatory response in acute stress-induced (Takotsubo) cardiomyopathy. JACC. Basic to Translational Science. 2018;**3**:766-778

[76] Surikow SY, Raman B, Licari J, et al. Evidence of nitrosative stress within hearts of patients dying of Takotsubo cardiomyopathy. International Journal of Cardiology. 2015;**189**:112-114

[77] Scally C, Abbas H, Ahearn T, et al. Myocardial and systemic inflammation

in acute stress-induced (Takotsubo) cardiomyopathy. Circulation. 2019;**139**:1581-1592

[78] Mueller KAL, Heinzmann D, Klingel K, et al. Histopathological and immunological characteristics of tachycardia-induced cardiomyopathy. Journal of the American College of Cardiology. 2017;**69**(17):2160-2172

[79] Farrell AS, Kuller JA, Goldstein SA, et al. Peripartum cardiomyopathy. Obstetrical & Gynecological Survey. 2021;**76**(8):485-492

[80] Bala R, Mehta S, Roy VC, et al. Peripartum cardiomyopathy: A review. Revista Portuguesa de Cardiologia. 2023;**42**(11):917-924

[81] Arany Z, Elkayam U. Peripartum cardiomyopathy. Circulation. 2016;**133**(14):1397-1409

[82] Hilfiker-Kleiner D, Kaminski K, Podewski E, et al. A cathepsin D-cleaved 16 kDa form of prolactin mediates postpartum cardiomyopathy. Cell. 2007;**128**(3):589-600

[83] Halkein J, Tabruyn SP, Ricke-Hoch M, et al. MicroRNA-146a is a therapeutic target and biomarker for peripartum cardiomyopathy. The Journal of Clinical Investigation. 2013;**123**(5):2143-2154

[84] Goli R, Li J, Brandimarto J, et al. Genetic and phenotypic landscape of peripartum cardiomyopathy. Circulation. 2021;**143**(19):1852-1862

[85] Liu J, Wang Y, Chen M, et al. The correlation between peripartum cardiomyopathy and autoantibodies against cardiovascular receptors. PLoS One. 2014;**9**(1):e86770

Chapter 2

Infiltrative Cardiomyopathies: Pathophysiology and Implications for Heart Transplantation

Ye In Christopher Kwon, Eleanor E. Bashian, Elizabeth J. Bashian, Justin Chang, Valentina Robila, Keyur B. Shah, Mohammed Makkiya and Zubair A. Hashmi

Abstract

Infiltrative cardiomyopathies may be an increasingly recognized, yet often overlooked, etiology of heart failure and cardiac arrhythmias, thus requiring a high degree of clinical suspicion. The appropriate utilization of various cardiac imaging plays a crucial role in the diagnosis and assessment of disease progression. This review aims to provide a comprehensive overview of the epidemiology, pathophysiology, clinical presentation, diagnosis, and treatment of ICM. We also highlight the current and upcoming medical and surgical management strategies for advanced ICM patients who present with heart failure and include a discussion surrounding orthotopic heart transplantation as a viable treatment option with curative intent.

Keywords: infiltrative cardiomyopathies, heart transplantation, amyloidosis, sarcoidosis, hemochromatosis

1. Introduction

Infiltrative cardiomyopathies (ICM) represent a diverse category of myocardial disorders distinguished by the deposition of anomalous cells, proteins, or molecules in myocardium [1]. Myocardial infiltration may manifest as extracellular or intracellular, the latter of which is better defined as a myocardial storage disorder [2]. Extracellular infiltration is best exemplified by cardiac amyloidosis whereas intracellular infiltration is seen in hemochromatosis [3]. In cardiac sarcoidosis, abnormal immune reactions can cause ICM characterized by noncaseating granulomatous infiltrations [4]. Rarely, hereditary conditions such as Fabry, Danon, Pompe disease, Friedreich Ataxia, Myocardial Oxalosis, and Mucopolysaccharidoses may also exhibit cardiac manifestations resulting in ICM [5]. In general, these infiltrative pathologies are thought to generate an inflammatory response progressing to fibrosis and increased wall thickening [6]. Diminished ventricular compliance results in notably increased left ventricular (LV) filling pressure, atrial enlargement, and congestion in both pulmonary and systemic veins. Consequently, such disease processes perpetuate irreversible tissue damage resulting in systolic and/or diastolic dysfunction, increased mechanical stress, microvascular dysfunction, and decreased coronary flow, potentially culminating in heart failure and premature mortality [1, 7].

ICM may be an increasingly recognized, yet often overlooked, etiology of heart failure and cardiac arrhythmias, thus requiring a high degree of clinical suspicion. The appropriate utilization of various cardiac imaging plays a crucial role in the diagnosis and assessment of disease progression [3]. This review aims to provide a comprehensive overview of the epidemiology, pathophysiology, clinical presentation, diagnosis, and treatment of ICM. We also highlight the current and upcoming medical and surgical management strategies for advanced ICM patients who present with heart failure and include a discussion surrounding orthotopic heart transplantation as a viable treatment option with curative intent.

2. Cardiac amyloidosis

Amyloidosis denotes the extracellular accumulation of fibrils made up of various serum proteins [8]. Factors that increase the likelihood of developing amyloidosis include older age, male sex, African descent, concurrent chronic ailments, and a family history, particularly in cases of inherited amyloidosis [9]. Several subtypes exist with similar molecular pathophysiology, but different precursor proteins, immunohistochemical features, genetics, prognosis, and therapeutic strategies [10]. These subtypes include primary amyloid light chain (AL), hereditary transthyretin-derived (hATTR; also known as familial amyloid cardiomyopathy), wild-type transthyretin-derived (wtATTR; also known as senile systemic), secondary (AA), and isolated atrial (AANF) amyloidosis [3, 10]. Despite advancements in cardiac imaging enabling earlier diagnosis, cardiac amyloidosis continues to have an unfavorable prognosis [11].

2.1 Epidemiology

The true prevalence of cardiac amyloidosis remains unknown. Over 95% of clinical cardiac amyloidosis stems from AL and ATTR [12, 13], with AL being the most common form of systemic amyloidosis. AL has a reported incidence of 1.2 per 100,000 with less than 50% cardiac involvement [14]. The absence of a dedicated diagnostic code for cardiac amyloidosis in the International Classification of Diseases, Ninth Revision (ICD-9), limits precise epidemiological data. Likewise, the prevalence of ATTR remains insufficiently explored. Recent evidence suggests that wtATTR may be underdiagnosed. The prevalence of wtATTR increases with age, particularly for those aged >80 years [15]. wtATTR has been identified in 13% of elderly patients hospitalized with heart failure and preserved ejection fraction (HFpEF) exhibiting increased wall thickness. Furthermore, TTR amyloid depositions are discovered postmortem in more than 30% of individuals over 75 years old with HFpEF. Recent data among hospitalized Medicare beneficiaries (2000–2014) demonstrate that cardiac amyloidosis is increasingly diagnosed among those over 65 years old who are hospitalized for HFpEF. Although the incidence was relatively similar between genders, cardiac amyloidosis prevalence was higher in men than women. It was around 2006 when a distinct inflection point became evident for both incident and prevalent cases of cardiac amyloidosis, with the most significant impact observed within the black population, regardless of gender, and notably in the age group >75 years [16]. Since ICD-10 has begun incorporating specific coding for cardiac amyloidosis, we may expect to challenge the notion that cardiac amyloidosis is a rare condition, particularly among elderly hospitalized patients.

2.2 Pathophysiology and clinical features

In cardiac amyloidosis, amyloid fibrils deposit in the extracellular myocardium. The culprit proteins are misfolded into antiparallel β-pleated sheets, conferring unique seeding activity and resistance to proteolysis [3, 17]. Amyloid deposition within the cardiac tissue disrupts both the mechanical contraction and electrical conduction, impacting coronary blood flow [3]. Initial stages may manifest as subtle diastolic impairments. However, as the disease progresses, there is a notable thickening of the cardiac wall characterized by a dense and elastic texture, leading to further deterioration in cardiac relaxation and compliance [18]. Consequently, diastolic filling pressures rise, leading to biventricular dysfunction and restrictive cardiomyopathy. As the atrium compensates, it leads to further atrial dilation [19]. Deposition of amyloid fibrils in key areas such as the sinoatrial (SA) and atrioventricular (AV) nodes, and bundle branches can give rise to varying degrees of heart block or ventricular arrhythmias [20]. Further damage to myocytes and localized fibrosis can also lead to systolic dysfunction [3]. Additionally, involvement of the distal coronary microvasculature can give rise to focal or diffuse areas of myocardial ischemia, further exacerbating myocardial dysfunction [21]. Although uncommon, obstructive intramural coronary amyloidosis can precipitate acute myocardial infarction [21, 22]. Recent evidence suggests that oxidative stress and toxicity, induced by misfolded light chain immunoglobulin, altered or misfolded TTR, and amyloid fibrils, may also play major roles in the pathogenesis of cardiac amyloidosis [22, 23].

Clinically significant heart failure due to cardiac amyloidosis may or may not occur concurrently with other symptoms of systemic amyloidosis. While dyspnea and exercise intolerance may be present, pulmonary edema is infrequent, with a predominance of symptoms indicating right-sided heart failure, such as lower extremity edema, hepatomegaly, and ascites [24]. Clinical symptoms, including angina and elevated troponin levels, may resemble acute coronary syndrome, even in the absence of coronary artery obstruction on angiography [18, 25, 26]. Syncope and presyncope may also occur, stemming from factors such as autonomic dysfunction, heightened sensitivity to intravascular fluid depletion within a restrictive physiological environment, and occasionally ventricular arrhythmias [27]. Advanced presentations may involve high-grade conduction abnormalities necessitating pacemaker placement, cardiac tamponade due to pericardial involvement, and systemic thromboembolism originating from atrial thrombi [28–30]. However, the pathophysiology of cardiac amyloidosis differs significantly by the variations in the precursor protein or molecules.

3. Primary light chain amyloidosis (AL)

AL is caused by a small clone of B-cells in the bone marrow that produces a light chain with mutations in the variable region. The LV1–44 gene is correlated with cardiac complications [31]. Mutations in this gene facilitate improper protein aggregation and misfolding, which drives primary organ dysfunction [32]. Cytotoxicity of cells are most prominently affected by the oligomers created from interactions with the extracellular milieu, including chaperones, matrix constituents, endoproteases, and various metallic elements [33]. Both misfolded proteins and oligomers have the capacity to trigger cellular stress, disturb tissue function, and worsen pathological transformations [34].

In cardiac AL, the pattern of light chain amyloid depositions is subendocardial and mostly diffuse [35]. Untreated prognosis is severe, with a median survival rate of less than one year [36]. The median survival of advanced stage cardiac AL is approximately 6 months [37]. Hypotension is common, and individuals with pre-existing hypertension may experience a decrease in blood pressure. Orthostatic hypotonia can also occur, particularly in the presence of autonomic nervous system amyloidosis. Additionally recurrent pleural effusions can be caused by cardiovascular failure in the context of amyloidosis and pleural amyloid infiltration [38]. As AL is predominantly a systemic disease, extracardiac manifestations may cue the clinician into making the initial diagnosis. Early in the disease process, nonspecific symptoms such as weakness, fatigue, and weight loss take precedence. Hepatomegaly arises due to liver infiltration or hepatic congestion. Renal involvement leads to significant proteinuria and the development of nephrotic syndrome. Purpura and easy bruising, particularly in the facial and neck regions, stem from deficiencies in clotting factors and delicate venules [3].

4. Hereditary transthyretin amyloidosis (hATTR)

hATTR is an autosomal dominant condition caused by more than 80 pathogenic mutations for the gene encoding the TTR protein [39]. The genetic alteration V122I is identified in approximately 3–4% of African descent individuals; however, its actual prevalence is often underestimated due to frequent misclassification as hypertensive cardiomyopathy [40]. TTR proteins are normally produced by the liver [41]. However, when pathologically aggregated into insoluble amyloid fibrils, the TTR deposits into the myocardium and peripheral nervous system to instigate irreversible neuropathy and cardiomyopathy. TTR amyloid fibrils infiltrate the interstitial spaces in the myocardium, resulting in stiffness and rigidity [42]. Myocardial fibrosis further impacts mechanical function of the heart, resulting in diastolic dysfunction from compromised ventricular compliance [42]. In advanced stages, hATTR cardiomyopathy occurs in up to 14% of patients with HFpEF [43, 44]. In patients with cardiac hATTR, persistently elevated left atrial pressures and dilatation can lead to atrial arrythmias [45]. Although ventricular arrhythmias have been documented in hATTR, they are notably less frequent than in AL cardiomyopathy [46].

Extra-cardiac manifestations of hATTR commonly affect the peripheral and autonomic nervous system. Progressively worsening peripheral neuropathy is often accompanied by hyperesthesia to pain, temperature dysregulation, motor weakness, and hypoactive tendon reflexes ascending from the lower extremities [3]. Furthermore, 13–21% of patients will develop lumbar spinal stenosis [47, 48]. Autonomic neuropathy related to hATTR features clinical symptoms including decreased bowel motility, incontinence, impotence, and orthostatic hypotension [49].

5. Wild-type transthyretin amyloidosis (wtATTR)

Also called senile systemic amyloidosis, wtATTR is considered to be an age-related process mostly affecting men >75 years old [50]. It has the capacity to affect not only cardiac tissues, but also the aorta, brain, lungs, pancreas, liver, and kidney [51].

The underlying mechanisms of pathogenesis remain poorly understood, with current theories suggesting the involvement of posttranslational modifications in the typically transcribed TTR or its associated chaperone proteins [52]. Autopsy data indicates that wtATTR is likely more common than previously thought, with 25% of male and female patients over 80 years old exhibiting evidence of TTR amyloid fibrils postmortem [53, 54]. This was corroborated by a prospective Finnish autopsy data involving 256 octogenarians, 25% of whom had wtATTR postmortem [53]. In a recent study, 86% of patients with wtATTR presented with diastolic heart failure or HFpEF with dyspnea on exertion, 64% with peripheral edema, and 67% with atrial fibrillation. In contrast to the nervous system manifestations in hATTR wtATTR is more commonly associated with cardiomyopathy. However, the wtATTR is also strongly associated with carpal tunnel syndrome. In the aforementioned study, 46% of patients exhibited a history of carpal tunnel syndrome, which may be an indicator of focal TTR accumulation that precedes cardiac manifestations by a number of years [42]. This finding aligns with another study that found approximately 10–16% of wtATTR patients reported carpal tunnel syndrome [55].

6. Secondary amyloidosis (AA)

Secondary amyloidosis (AA) is characterized by the deposition of amyloid A fibrils, an acute phase reactant protein [10]. AA is commonly associated with other chronic inflammatory conditions including rheumatoid arthritis, familial Mediterranean fever, chronic tuberculosis, and inflammatory bowel disease [56]. Cardiac manifestations of AA are thought to be exceedingly rare, occurring in less than 5% of cases [10, 56]. AA predominantly affects the kidneys, leading to proteinuria and ultimately, renal failure [57]. Importantly, the cardiac manifestations of AA can be reversed through appropriate treatment of the underlying disorder.

7. Isolated atrial amyloidosis (AANF)

AANF is characterized by the release of atrial natriuretic peptide (ANP) from the atrial myocytes when triggered by increased atrial wall distension. While 90% of AANF cases occur in female patients in their 90s, this condition can also occur in younger patients with valvular disease or in those with chronic atrial fibrillation. Pathologically, ANP fibrils are limited to the endocardium, presenting as thin, linear deposits along or just beneath [3, 58–62] the endocardium. The clinical relevance of this disease process remains unclear.

7.1 Diagnosis

The workup for patients with suspected cardiac amyloidosis includes electrocardiogram (ECG), echocardiogram, cardiac magnetic resonance imaging (CMR) and tissue biopsy. ECG may demonstrate low voltage QRS and AV blocks. Echocardiogram may show right and/or left ventricular hypertrophy, a granular speckled myocardium, or restricted basal longitudinal strain [1, 13]. CMR will demonstrate global or partial late gadolinium enhancement (LGE), although no specific pattern is diagnostic. Cine steady-state free precession images commonly exhibit concentric thickening of the myocardial wall, dilation of both atria, and impaired function of both ventricles [1].

The presence of amyloid deposition significantly modifies the behavior of gadolinium in the myocardium and blood pool. The elevated concentration of gadolinium in the extracellular compartment leads to a decrease in myocardial T1 relaxation time, while the rapid elimination of gadolinium from the blood pool prolongs the T1 relaxation time of the blood pool [63].

Cardiac scintigraphy utilizing bone-avid radiotracers can confirm the diagnosis of ATTR, eliminating the need for biopsy. Furthermore, the advancement of innovative tracers and the utilization of quantitative analysis hold promise for enhancing earlier detection of cardiac amyloidosis, improving the differentiation of cardiac amyloidosis subtypes, and assessing amyloid burden for prognostic purposes and evaluation of therapy response [12, 64, 65]. Importantly, a novel scoring system for ATTR cardiomyopathy, incorporating both clinical and echocardiographic parameters, could assist in the targeted identification of individuals with HFpEF who would benefit from undergoing cardiac scintigraphy. A score equal to or greater than six serves to isolate patients who are at a heightened risk for ATTR cardiac amyloidosis, displaying a commendable level of sensitivity and negative predictive value [1, 66].

Serum and urinary free light chain measurements, along with immunofixation electrophoresis, are valuable diagnostic tools for quantifying and identifying monoclonal proteins, respectively. These tests help in distinguishing AL amyloidosis from other forms by detecting abnormal light chains produced by clonal plasma cells. Quantifying free light chains in serum and urine can provide crucial information about the burden of amyloidogenic light chains and aid in monitoring disease progression and response to therapy. In general, patients may be worked up for unclear etiology as initial symptoms tend to be nonspecific. Endomyocardial biopsy can provide definitive diagnosis and should be considered if the patient is undergoing cardiac surgery or catheterization for another reason [67].

Micromorphologically, there are four patterns of amyloid deposits observable on hematoxylin and eosin staining, which can also coexist: interstitial, nodular, endocardial, and vascular. The interstitial or perimyocyte pattern is the most common in cardiac amyloidosis, often mimicking interstitial fibrosis. The amyloid deposits typically appear eosinophilic, amorphous, and homogeneous, predominantly located in extracellular space. They are frequently associated with cracking artifacts between the myocytes and amyloid, cardiomyocyte hypertrophy, and can be readily identified using special stains such as Congo Red and Sulfated Alcian Blue. Mass spectrometry of the tissue sample is indicated for typing the specific amyloid protein. Fine needle aspiration of the abdominal fat pad can also be utilized for tissue biopsy, which is generally safer and more feasible than endomyocardial biopsy [2, 10].

7.2 Management

Treatment strategies can be stratified into three areas: management of heart failure that occurs due to a restrictive cardiomyopathy by using standard heart failure management, management of arrhythmias through either medical therapy or device therapy and targeting the underlying protein disorder via disease modifying agents. In AL, immunotherapy may be used to target the B cells which are responsible for producing the misfolding light chains. The ANDROMEDA trial investigated adding daratumumab, an anti-CD38 antibody, to conventional treatment. Daratumumab is an anti-CD38 antibody that induces cell death. The results have been promising with a 3-fold higher likelihood of complete hematologic response in patients treated with both [68]. On the other hand, bortezomib induces apoptosis of rapidly dividing cells by inhibiting the proteasome and preventing activation of NFkB [69]. Following this trial, daratumumab and bortezomib have become standard [41, 70, 71].

ATTR is treated with diflunisal (non-steroidal anti-inflammatory [NSAID]) and tafamidis (non-NSAID [10]). In the double-blind, multicenter randomized control trial ATTR-ACT, the efficacy of tafamidis, a benzoxazole derivative that stabilizes mutant TTR tetramers, was evaluated. In addition to reducing all-cause mortality (29.5 vs. 42.9%,; hazard ratio: 0.7, 95% Confidence Interval [CI]: 0.51 to 0.96) and cardiovascular-related hospitalizations (0.48 per year vs. 0.70 per year, 95% CI: 0.56 to 0.81), patients treated with tafamidis also experience less decline in functional capacity, measured by 6-minute walk test, and quality of life, measured by scores on the Kansas City Cardiomyopathy Questionnaire Overall Summary (KCQQ-OS [72, 73]). Despite its efficacy in delaying disease progression, the high cost of tafamidis ($200,000 per year) restricts its widespread use [71]. As an alternative, diflunisal is a NSAID that acts as a tetramer stabilizer. In a meta-analysis of six studies with a total of 400 patients, it was largely shown to slow disease progression and preserve quality of life [74].

7.3 Implications for heart transplantation

Numerous case series involving consecutive orthotopic heart transplantation (OHT) and autologous stem cell transplantation (ASCT) have investigated the role of heart transplantation for patients with advanced cardiac amyloidosis. However, the prognosis for patients with AL amyloidosis undergoing cardiac transplantation in the absence of sequential ASCT is unfavorable, with a limited 3- to 5-year survival rate [75–77]. Conversely, sequential OHT-ASCT enhances survival outcomes at the 1-year mark. Thus, some centers have decided to implement a waiting period of at least 1 year post-OHT before proceeding to ASCT, a management strategy which differs from previous small case series, which suggested waiting times ranging from 6 to 9 months between OHT and ASCT [78]. Notably, this has not resulted in amyloid disease recurrence in the transplanted heart or clinically significant dysfunction of the cardiac allograft [78]. Nevertheless, there's a risk of patients experiencing partial remission post-ASCT which may necessitate a kidney transplant due to the progression of amyloid-related kidney complications [78].

There are several key elements to consider when evaluating cardiac amyloidosis patients for OHT or ASCT. The major risk factor associated with OHT in patients with end-stage cardiac amyloidosis is the involvement of other major organs, such as the recurrence in the cardiac allograft resulting in reduced 1- and 5-year post-transplant survival rates [79, 80]. Early transplantation cases in the United Kingdom, involving 24 individuals (predominantly due to AL amyloidosis) devoid of supplementary chemotherapy, exhibited distressing 1- and 5-year survival rates of 50 and 20%, respectively [79]. While overall 1- and 5-year survival for OHT remains 89 and 75%, respectively, OHT for cardiac amyloidosis has historically been linked with inferior post-transplant survival rates [81]. Nevertheless, the introduction of light-chain reductive chemotherapy and post-heart-transplant autologous hematopoietic stem cell transplant (ASCT) has enhanced the post-heart-transplant prognosis for patients with cardiac amyloidosis. Drawing from the United Kingdom's experience, post-heart-transplant reductive chemotherapy has raised the survival rate to 71% at 1 year [79]. A recent study out of Stanford also demonstrated that while patients with cardiac AL and ATTR were older and had longer waitlist times, rates of postoperative survival, bleeding, renal failure, infection, rejection or malignancy did not differ when compared to non-amyloidosis patients [82]. Furthermore, in hATTR, heart transplant alone may not prevent the progressively disabling polyneuropathy. It is recommended that for these patients, concomitant liver transplant should be considered with curative intent. Nevertheless, in the contemporary period of potent pharmacological treatments, the necessity of liver transplantation remains ambiguous, especially when compared to an alternative strategy involving OHT alongside pharmacotherapy. Prior to carrying out OHT in individuals with mutations linked to mixed-phenotype disorder, conducting a comprehensive neurological assessment to rule out clinically substantial neuropathy is imperative [83].

Cardiac amyloidosis patients, especially those with AL, face a significant mortality risk while awaiting transplantation, ranging from 24 to 40% [84, 85]. The 2018 modifications to the heart allocation system acknowledged this elevated mortality risk by assigning amyloidosis patients a higher status (status 4) on the transplant list. Notably, there is no distinction between AL and ATTR amyloidosis in this allocation criteria, as amyloidosis is categorized alongside hypertrophic and other restrictive cardiomyopathies [86]. Preliminary data indicates improved transplantation rates and reduced waiting list mortality for individuals with infiltrative cardiomyopathy following these adjustments [87]. While OHT poses significant challenges in systemic or cardiac amyloidosis, careful patient selection with focus on effective pharmacotherapies before and after transplantation can yield acceptable outcomes.

7.4 Future directions

The landscape of treatment for cardiac amyloidosis is changing rapidly. In general, treatment has been aimed at stopping production of misfolded protein; however, there exists an unmet need to target already deposited amyloid fibrils. Two treatments are under investigation. Doxycycline was found to disrupt fibril formation and prevent amyloid deposition in transgenic mouse models [88–90]. Subsequently, a retrospective analysis of patients with cardiac AL revealed higher hematologic response and better survival in patients treated with doxycycline [91]. However, when evaluated in a randomized control trial, no benefit was observed. In this multicenter trial, 140 patients with Mayo 2004 stage II to III light chain amyloidosis were randomized to 100 mg doxycycline twice daily with CyBorD (9 cycles) or CyBorD (9 cycles) alone. No improvement in 2-year progression-free survival was observed [69].

The second treatment under investigation is Birtamimab, a humanized IgG1 that targets misfolded light chains to promote phagocytic clearance of AL deposits [92]. In a double-blind randomized control trial, VITAL, patients were treated with 24 mg/kg Birtamimab plus standard of care or placebo plus standard of care every 28 days [92]. This study was terminated early following an interim futility analysis. However, a follow-up study, AFFIRM-AL (A Study to Evaluate the Efficacy and Safety of Birtamimab in Mayo Stage IV Patients with AL Amyloidosis) is currently enrolling only patients with more advanced forms of cardiac AL amyloidosis based on post-hoc analysis of VITAL results [93].

Another promising therapeutic agent, CAEL-101, is in the developmental pipeline. CAEL-101 is an amyloid fibril–reactive chimeric immunoglobulin G1k monoclonal antibody. Upon binding to misfolded light chains, CAEL-101 triggers the activation of neutrophils and initiates a proteolytic cascade directed against AL fibrils. Encouraging findings from a recent phase 1a/b trial involving CAEL-101 in patients with relapsed or refractory AL-CA lend support to the notion that this agent may enhance target organ function by improving the LV global longitudinal strain and reducing NT-proBNP levels following a 12-week treatment period [94]. We eagerly wait for the data from a phase 3 trial testing the effect of CAEL-101 on the outcomes of newly diagnosed cardiac AL cases.

The role of RNA silencers is also emerging. These agents function by suppressing TTR synthesis in the liver, effectively eliminating the necessity for liver transplantation. Various agents have been on trial for patients suffering from hATTR-related polyneuropathy, including inotersen, patisiran, and vutrisiran. These have shown significant improvements in neuropathy impairment scores for hATTR patients [95–97]. However, the cost of these agents, averaging around $450,000 per year, pose a significant barrier to access [98]. The role of RNA silencers in cardiac ATTR remains to be seen, as we await the results of a randomized controlled trial with PRX004 [99]. Furthermore, there are therapies in development aimed at prevention of amyloid cardiomyopathy among those who carry the pathogenic mutations. In this arena, gene-editing by CRISPR-CAS9 may represent the future therapy for cardiac amyloidosis. NTLA 2001, developed by Intellia Therapeutics and Regeneron Pharmaceuticals, represents a CRISPR-CAS9–based in vivo gene editing platform. This innovative technology has displayed potential as a viable treatment option during the initial phase of clinical testing in individuals suffering from ATTR polyneuropathy [100]. The potential promise of CRISPR-CAS9 may offer a definitive cure for patients with genetic predisposition to hATTR.

8. Cardiac sarcoidosis

Sarcoidosis is a systemic granulomatous condition with an uncertain etiology [101]. Current evidence suggests that it arises from an immunological reaction to an unidentified antigenic stimulus in genetically predisposed individuals [102]. The characteristic histopathological feature is noncaseating granulomas. The lungs are impacted in over 90% of cases, with potential involvement of other organs such as the heart, liver, spleen, skin, eyes, parotid gland, and various tissues. The majority of cases (70%) are diagnosed in individuals aged between 25 and 60 years, while occurrences in those below 15 or above 70 years are infrequent [103]. Sarcoidosis exhibits a global distribution, with prevalence ranging from 4.7 to 64 per 100,000 individuals [101]. Notably, higher incidence rates are documented among northern European and African American populations, particularly affecting women [104, 105].

The presence of familial clusters underscores a significant hereditary component in sarcoidosis [106]. However, the interplay between genetic and environmental factors, including organ-specificity, remains unknown. Clinically significant cardiac involvement occurs in approximately 5% of sarcoidosis patients, although approximately 25% of patients with systemic sarcoidosis display asymptomatic or clinically silent cardiac participation [107, 108]. Underdiagnosis and lack of reliable reference standards worsen prognosis. Cardiac sarcoidosis is associated with mortality resulting from ventricular arrhythmias, high degree heart block, and heart failure [1].

8.1 Epidemiology

Studies indicate that there is a growing prevalence of cardiac sarcoidosis, likely due to advancements in diagnostic imaging. The diagnostic rate of cardiac sarcoidosis in Finland surged by over 20 times between 1988 and 2012 [109, 110]. Similarly, in the United States, the proportion of transplant recipients with cardiac sarcoidosis-induced cardiomyopathy escalated from 0.1% (1994 to 1997) to 0.5%

(2010 to 2014 [111]). Incidence and prevalence of cardiac sarcoidosis varies widely by regions. Scandinavian countries are thought to have the highest incidence with an estimated 11.5 cases per 100,00. In contrast, the United States has an incidence rate between 8 and 11 cases per 100,000. East Asian countries, particularly South Korea, have some of the lowest incidence at 0.5–1.3 cases per 100,000 [112]. Sarcoidosis is not commonly considered an age-related condition. Rather, it typically occurs in patients aged 25 to 45 years, with women aged older than 50 years being the most affected population in Japan and European countries [113].

There are also notable racial and ethnic disparities in cardiac sarcoidosis. An examination of a national healthcare database in the United States spanning from 2010 to 2013 demonstrated a prevalence rate among Black Americans (141.4 per 100,00) that was three times greater than that of White Americans (49.8 per 100,00). Conversely, Hispanics and Asians exhibited a lower prevalence at 21.7 per 100,000 and 18.9 per 100,000, respectively. Notably, the highest prevalence was observed in Black American women, reaching 178.5 per 100,000 [114]. The Black Women's Health Study projected an average annual incidence rate of up to 71 per 100,000 among Black American women, with a prevalence rate nearing 2%. [115] Moreover, an increased mortality rate was documented among women and Black Americans [116].

While sarcoidosis most commonly affects the lungs, there is growing recognition that cardiac sarcoidosis may be its first manifestation [117]. A significant proportion of individuals, ranging from 16 to 35%, who present with complete AV block (age < 60 years) or VT of unknown origin, are subsequently discovered to have undiagnosed cardiac sarcoidosis [118, 119]. The detection of cardiac sarcoidosis as the primary etiology of heart failure is frequently overlooked; a notable example being the identification of previously undiagnosed cardiac sarcoidosis in 6 out of 177 patients through core LV biopsies conducted during left ventricular assist device (LVAD) insertion [120].

8.2 Pathophysiology and clinical features

Cardiac sarcoidosis is characterized by granulomatous infiltration that disrupts normal organ function. It is characterized by three successive stages: edema, granuloma formation, and fibrosis [10]. The instigating antigenic trigger remains unclear. However, several factors have been proposed, including genetic predisposition, prior infections, and environmental exposures. Human leukocyte antigen (HLA) alleles in the major histocompatibility complex genes such as the HLA DQB*0601 and the TNFA2 allele are associated with cardiac sarcoidosis in Japanese women [121, 122]. In addition, HLA-DR17(3) displays the strongest correlation with sarcoidosis within the White demographic. Meanwhile, chronic disease progression is linked to HLA-DR15(2) or DR14(6) [123]. Major infectious agents include mycobacterium, Propionibacterium, *Borrelia burgdorferi*, *Rickettsia helvetica*, Epstein–Barr virus, and the human herpes virus [124]. Interestingly, there have been reports of sarcoidosis related to occupational exposures [116].

Following exposure to these agents, sarcoid development is predominantly driven by an exaggerated TH1 cell reaction leading to the secretion of various cytokines such as interleukin (IL)-2, interferon γ, and IL-12. This initial phase is succeeded by an anti-inflammatory TH2 response characterized by the presence of IL-4, IL-5, IL-10, and IL-13 cytokines [125]. The formation and resolution of cardiac granulomas correspond to the presence of these cytokines in a specific sequence [126]. The fibrotic transition is facilitated by the shift towards a TH2 response, aided by platelet-derived growth factor-B, insulin-like growth factor 1, and insulin-like growth factor binding protein-related protein 2 [127, 128]. Recent research also highlights the involvement of IFN-γ producing Th17 cells in the pathogenesis of sarcoidosis and proposes discrepancies in Tregs and Th17 cell response [127, 129].

In cardiac sarcoidosis, the myocardium, endocardium, or epicardium are involved extensively [126, 130, 131]. Granulomas are commonly seen in the basal interventricular septum, LV wall, and more rarely, atria [132–134]. As the disease advances, the granulomatous inflammation triggers a repair response that manifests with scarring, which is notably different from those observed in myocardial infarction. Sarcoidosis-related scarring appears more patchy, rather than extensive, in the subendocardial or transmural regions [126]. The presence of granulomas in the interventricular septum can lead to conduction blocks that may respond to steroid treatment, whereas patchy scarring of the myocardium creates a focal point for ventricular tachyarrhythmias, focal aneurysms, and both systolic and diastolic dysfunction of the left ventricle (LV), eventually perpetuating heart failure [128].

The clinical presentation of sarcoidosis depends on the stage of disease. At the edema stage, diastolic dysfunction occurs. As sarcoidosis progresses to granuloma formation, global or segmental hypokinesia presents. Finally, systolic dysfunction is observed with fibrosis [125]. In general, screening is only recommended for symptomatic patients with known sarcoidosis, as these patients are at higher risk for heart failure, ventricular dysrhythmias, and sudden cardiac death [135]. In patients with no diagnosis of sarcoidosis, sustained monomorphic ventricular tachycardias, second- or third-degree heart block in young individuals, new onset cardiomyopathy or heart failure, or unexplained wall motion abnormalities or wall thinning should raise suspicion for cardiac sarcoidosis. Several presentations can be seen: (i) conduction abnormalities including bundle branch or AV block, (ii) ventricular arrhythmias which can include sudden death, palpitations, dizziness, syncope, (iii) heart failure manifesting as the standard constellation of CHF symptoms (DOE, orthopnea, etc.), or (iv) silent disease in which pulmonary or systemic symptoms are primary findings but imaging findings demonstrate cardiac involvement [125, 128, 136].

8.3 Diagnosis

Initial evaluation starts with imaging. ECG findings will often show dysrhythmias and high-grade block, and echocardiograms can show septal thinning or thickening; segmental wall motion abnormalities may also be seen [137]. CMR offers superior spatial resolution, capability to offer tissue characterization, and concurrent structural and functional evaluation of the myocardium [138, 139]. The distinctive phases of acute and chronic cardiac sarcoidosis can be distinguished through various technical components of CMR. LGE stands out as the most dependable tool in the evaluation of cardiac sarcoidosis using CMR [117]. There is no definitive distribution pattern indicative of cardiac sarcoidosis, however research suggests LGE predominantly in the subepicardial or mid-myocardial regions of the basal septum and LV lateral wall with possible extension into the right ventricle may indicate cardiac sarcoidosis [133, 140, 141]. Occasionally, LGE may present as subendocardial, resembling an infarction pattern [140]. While LGE aids in identifying more chronic stages associated with fibrosis or scarring, T2 mapping can detect elevated water content or edema in regions with active inflammation. Furthermore, positron emission tomography (PET) may be a valuable tool in cardiac sarcoidosis, given that 18F-FDG accumulates in inflammatory cells within the hearts of affected individuals [1].

There is no specific pathognomonic pattern for FDG uptake for cardiac sarcoidosis [142]. Current evidence suggests that FDG-PET appears to possess greater sensitivity but lower specificity than CMR, and its utility is most evident in patients for whom CMR is contraindicated or unavailable [1, 143]. The dual use of CMR and FDG-PET may offer superior diagnostic value.

Myocardial biopsy is considered the gold standard and may demonstrate hallmark histopathology; however, extracardiac biopsy can also be considered due to improved safety profile [10]. Histological examination of the heart in cardiac sarcoidosis reveals non-necrotizing, epithelioid granulomas, with or without multinucleated giant cells, that can involve all layers of the heart. A common diagnostic challenge is differentiating cardiac sarcoidosis from giant cell myocarditis, as both conditions exhibit overlapping histologic features. Giant cell myocarditis is characterized by diffuse mixed inflammatory infiltrates with prominent multinucleated giant cells, but unlike cardiac sarcoidosis, these giant cells are associated with adjacent myocyte necrosis and do not form distinct granulomas. Additionally, in giant cell myocarditis, the giant cells do not involve the epicardium or pericardial fat, which can be seen in cardiac sarcoidosis. Due to the heterogeneous myocardial involvement in cardiac sarcoidosis, myocardial biopsy is highly specific but not sensitive, detecting sarcoidosis in only 20–50% of cases. Moreover, since cardiac sarcoidosis may present with scattered giant cells in areas lacking well-formed granulomas, distinguishing it from giant cell myocarditis based on biopsy specimens alone can be particularly challenging.

Clinically, several sets of diagnostic criteria have been proposed although none have been widely adopted. The Japanese Ministry of Health and Wealthware (JMHW) proposed both a histological (i.e., biopsy confirmed) and a clinical route to diagnosis [144]. Clinical diagnosis involves a histologic diagnosis of extracardiac sarcoidosis along with cardiac symptoms meeting major and minor criteria [144]. The World Association of Sarcoidosis and Other Granulomatous diseases (WASOG) Organ Assessment Instrument is a clinical tool which utilizes expert opinion to determine the likelihood of organ involvement based on three categories [145]. However, neither of these tools have been validated in large cohorts and there is generally a lack of consensus on best practices for accurate diagnosis. Early identification before scar formation can lead to better outcomes with treatment. The extent of myocardial involvement and ventricular dysrhythmias upon presentation also affect prognosis [146].

8.4 Management

The goal of medical management for cardiac sarcoidosis is to reduce the inflammation and limit the development of myocardial fibrosis [128]. Treatment relies on multiple modalities of immunosuppression, including corticosteroids, disease modifying agents, and biologics. The survival benefit of corticosteroids in sarcoidosis has not yet been proven in a randomized controlled trial [147]. The most reliable data pertained to the efficacy of corticosteroids in patients with AV block. However, glucocorticoids continue to be the mainstay of first-line treatment. Patient input and close follow-up is paramount to determine the optimal doses and regimen. It is recommended that the initial dosage range from 30 to 40 mg/day [10, 148] and that treatment response be assessed within 1 to 3 months [10]. If the patient responds positively, the steroid dosage should be gradually reduced to 5 to 15 mg/day for an additional 9 to 12 months [148]. Patients should be monitored for a minimum of 3 years post-treatment cessation to detect potential relapses [103].

Second-line treatments for cardiac sarcoidosis include cytolytic agents such as nucleotide analogs and precursor analogs [149], some of which include methotrexate (MTX), a folate antagonist, or azathioprine, an antagonist of purine metabolism [149]. MTX, in particular, is frequently employed as a secondary option in cases of treatment resistance and/or in the presence of adverse effects from steroids [150]. Mycophenolate mofetil and azathioprine, two antimetabolite agents, are also increasingly utilized as treatment options [149]. Other agents include azathioprine, cyclophosphamide, and infliximab [101]. There is not yet a consensus on whether corticosteroids should be universally administered to all cardiac sarcoidosis patients or reserved only for those displaying specific clinical symptoms.

TNFa blockers and inhibitors are third-line or alternative treatments [149]. In small trials, infliximab, a monoclonal anti-TNF-alpha antibody, has been shown to be effective in refractory cases. If medically refractory, ventricular assist devices (VAD) or other forms of mechanical circulatory support can be used as destination therapy or bridge to transplant. Primary transplantation may also be considered [128].

8.5 Implications for heart transplantation

Despite medical management, patients may eventually develop heart failure from cardiac sarcoidosis [149, 151, 152]. A recent study from Finland found that 14% of patients with clinically manifested cardiac sarcoidosis progressed to advanced heart failure within 15 years of diagnosis, despite medical management [153]. LV ejection fraction (LVEF) <50% and elevated cardiac troponins predicted 25% of 15-year risk of end-stage heart failure [153]. Thus, advanced heart failure treatments such as durable mechanical support or OHT should be carefully evaluated [154, 155]. Factors to consider include the extent of extracardiac sarcoidosis and other organ involvement, which may impact post-transplant mortality and morbidity [128]. Pre-existing immunosuppression-related complications including diabetes, susceptibility to adrenal insufficiency, and impaired wound healing should also be considered [149].

Outcomes of OHT in patients with cardiac sarcoidosis have been similar to those with other cardiomyopathies [156]. A 2018 analysis of the United Network for Organ Sharing (UNOS) database found 91 and 83% survival at 1- and 5-year intervals, respectively, for cardiac sarcoidosis patients, compared to 90 and 77% for other recipients at same time intervals [155]. Importantly, patients with cardiac sarcoidosis undergoing OHT had lower odds of organ rejection compared to non-cardiac patients [156]. In cases where the consideration of an LV assist device (LVAD) arises, it is crucial to assess the level of the RV involvement, arrhythmic, and infection risks associated with immunosuppression. For instance, conditions such as predominant RV failure, restrictive cardiomyopathy, or a high burden of ventricular arrhythmias may not respond well to durable LVAD therapy, necessitating tailored bridge-to-transplantation approaches that involve biventricular mechanical support.

There continues to be a lack of data on long-term outcomes of LVADs or OHT in patients with cardiac sarcoidosis. However, it is worth noting that because cardiac sarcoidosis is often undetected until examination of the native heart tissue during LVAD or OHT, there is likely some degree of clinical misclassification prior to surgery [157]. Collaboration between multidisciplinary sarcoidosis teams and advanced heart failure specialists is critical for patients with cardiac sarcoidosis undergoing OHT or LVAD support.

8.6 Future directions

One of the major challenges in clinical trials for cardiac sarcoidosis has been non standardized and unguided endpoints. WASOG convened in 2011 to generate standardized trial endpoint recommendations based on clinical manifestations and symptoms [158]. While progress has been made in recent trials to meet clear primary endpoints, most trials have not met task force recommendations for those endpoints [159]. Moreover, enhancing reporting uniformity may aid in result interpretation and better convey the progress of therapeutic pipelines to patients. Despite these challenges, several recent trials merit discussion. In the Cardiac Sarcoidosis multi-center randomized controlled trial (CHASM-CS), low-dose prednisone-MTX combination therapy was compared to prednisone alone with varying doses and duration of treatment; outcomes from this trial have not yet been published [160]. Notably, the PRESTIGE study recently found no significant differences in the efficacy of methotrexate or a second dose of prednisolone in patients with cardiac sarcoidosis who did not respond to initial prednisolone therapy. This is a particularly important concept that provides evidence to the utility of methotrexate as a potential steroid-sparing agent. However, further studies are needed to assess the therapeutic efficacy of methotrexate in cardiac sarcoidosis, including its precise mechanism of action when administered at higher dosages or for extended durations.

9. Cardiac hemochromatosis

Iron overload cardiomyopathies (IOC) arise due to abnormalities in iron homeostasis that are attributed to either hereditary or acquired etiologies. Primary IOC, also known as cardiac hemochromatosis, stems from a mutation in the HFE gene typically inherited in an autosomal recessive manner [161]. These patients often present asymptomatic in the early stages, further complicating prevention and diagnosis. Thus, patients with cardiac hemochromatosis will often have damage in other organs related to excess iron by the time of diagnosis [162]. Conversely, secondary causes of IOC encompass hemoglobinopathies and myelodysplastic syndromes (MDS) [1]. The extent of cardiac involvement varies on the specific etiology. Thalassemia patients experience prominently high mortality due to heart failure [162]. In comparison, heart disease does not appear to be a large cause of mortality and morbidity among sickle cell patients [163].

The infiltration and deposition of iron is believed to begin in the epicardium before diffusing throughout the myocardium and endocardium [164]. The entire conduction system, particularly the AV node, is vulnerable to excess iron deposition [165]. Chronic iron overload can progressively lead to heart failure and arrhythmias. Therefore, cardiac hemochromatosis should be carefully considered in any patients with unexplained heart failure.

9.1 Epidemiology

Exact incidence and prevalence of cardiac hemochromatosis or primary IOC is unknown. However, it is estimated that in the United States roughly 1 in 300 Caucasian people have hereditary hemochromatosis [166]. In contrast, Northern Europeans have a substantially higher burden of disease as 1 in 15 individuals carry at least one variant of the HFE gene [167]. Hemochromatosis does not exhibit sex specificity; however, a higher proportion of males demonstrate symptoms and show an elevated risk of hepatic injury. In contrast, females may manifest hemochromatosis symptoms later in life because of regular blood loss during menstrual cycles [166, 168]. The epidemiology of secondary IOC can only be extrapolated by the prevalence and incidence of the differing underlying causes. For example, thalassemia is the most prominent cause of cardiac iron overload due to the need for frequent blood transfusions to correct their anemia. The global incidence of thalassemia is estimated to be 4.4 out of every 10,000 births. Alpha-thalassemia predominates among individuals of Southeast Asian descent. Beta-thalassemia, on the other hand, is most prevalent among populations with origins in the Mediterranean, Africa, and South Asia [165].

9.2 Pathophysiology and clinical features

Several subtypes of hereditary hemochromatosis exist. Type 1 makes up 80% of hemochromatosis and is caused by the HFE gene mutation on chromosome 6. Hepatic complications are most prominent in type 1. Type 2 is linked to mutations in the HJV gene located on chromosome 1, responsible for encoding hemojuvelin (subtype 2A), or in the HAMP gene on chromosome 19, which encodes hepcidin (subtype 2B). Cardiac manifestations, especially heart failure before the age of 30, are most seen in type 2. Type 3 arises from mutations in the TfR2 gene on chromosome 7, which encodes transferrin receptor 2. Conversely, type 4 is the result of mutations in the SLC40A1 gene on chromosome 2, which encodes ferroportin [169]. In contrast, secondary IOC primarily stems from the substantial administration of parenteral iron related to transfusion-dependent anemias. These include inherited hemoglobinopathies, MDS, myelofibrosis, aplastic anemia, sideroblastic anemia, and Blackfan-Diamond anemia [170]. In the case of inherited hemoglobinopathies, all patients with thalassemia major and approximately 20% of sickle cell patients require transfusions [171]. Similarly, a significant proportion of MDS patients now undergo chronic transfusions. Almost 50% of patients with MDS who receive 75–100 units of blood will develop clinically significant myocardial iron overload [171–173].

Myocardial iron uptake progresses at a slower rate hepatic uptake, leading to a delayed onset of myocardial iron overload in contrast to hepatic iron overload [170]. Iron accumulation initiates in the ventricular myocardium, extends to the atrial myocardium, and impacts the conducting system [170]. Although epicardial iron levels usually surpass subendocardial levels, a study indicates a consistent iron distribution across the LV in severe IOC patients [174]. Within myocytes, presence of excess labile iron triggers the production of reactive oxygen species, leading to the conversion of ferrous to ferric iron and the generation of the harmful hydroxyl radical, which overwhelms the antioxidant defenses. Concurrently, elevated ferrous iron transport through L-type calcium channels disrupts cardiomyocyte calcium handling. This affects excitation-contraction coupling and potentially contributes to the development of diastolic and systolic ventricular dysfunction leading to heart failure [173, 175]. It is important to note that in addition to myocardial iron overload, various immunoinflammatory and genetic factors appeared to influence the development of IOC, including myocarditis, the HLA genotype, and the apolipoprotein E genotype [173, 174, 176].

As with other forms of ICMs, the level of cardiac impairment is highly dependent on the severity of iron deposition in the myocardium. However, in general, there are two major clinical features of cardiac hemochromatosis. First, IOC-related dilated cardiomyopathy is characterized by LV enlargement and decreased LVEF [173].

Second, IOC can also cause restrictive cardiomyopathy and may present with exertional dyspnea. This process likely begins with diastolic LV dysfunction causing restrictive filling and increased filling pressures. While these patients may have preserved LVEF, they often progress to biventricular failure, which causes pulmonary hypertension, peripheral edema, and hepatic congestion [177]. These phenotypes often accompany a spectrum of other clinical manifestations including myocarditis, paroxysmal atrial fibrillation, ventricular arrhythmias, and atrial or ventricular tachyarrhythmias [178–180]. Notably, features of ischemic heart disease of myocardial infarction do not appear to be prominently associated with cardiac hemochromatosis [181].

9.3 Diagnosis

Echocardiography is the main modality of choice for evaluating potential heart failure patients with IOC [176]. Early observations include diastolic LV dysfunction and left atrial enlargement. In later stages, there's no notable dilatation of both the LV and RV and significantly reduced LVEF [164]. Alternatively, there may also be restrictive filling of the LV with dilatation of the left atrium and RV. In these cases, pulmonary artery pressures are likely elevated with preserved EF. The major limitation with regards to echocardiography is that it gives limited information about the actual myocardial iron content. Therefore, it is more often used as the primary screening tool for asymptomatic patients or for monitoring patients with established hereditary or acquired IOC [173].

CMR T2 analysis is the modality of choice for noninvasive, qualitative analysis of myocardial iron load, measured as hemosiderin, with high sensitivity and consistency [182]. There's some evidence that T1 may be more sensitive than T2 [183]. Therefore, recent guidelines recommend combined use of both T1 and T2 for improved sensitivity.

The importance of basic laboratory investigations merits further discussion in evaluation of IOC. These include serum ferritin, transferrin, full blood count, hemoglobin electrophoresis, liver function tests, and a comprehensive set of endocrine tests aimed at assessing the underlying etiology of IOC [173]. As with any hereditary conditions, genetic testing may also be considered for various hemoglobinopathies and hereditary hemochromatosis [184]. Furthermore, since hepatic iron uptake precedes myocardial iron deposition, liver biopsy may be performed before endomyocardial biopsy in patients with suspected IOC [184].

9.4 Management

Therapeutic phlebotomy is a safe and cost effective first-line treatment for all types of hereditary hemochromatosis, generally recommended for symptomatic patients with serum ferritin greater than 1000 ng/mL [173]. It involves an induction phase aimed at removing 1–2 units of blood per week to achieve a reduction of serum ferritin by <50 ng/mL and transferrin saturation < 30%. This is often followed by a life-long maintenance phase aimed at serum ferritin <100 ng/mL and transferrin saturation < 50% [173]. The downsides of phlebotomy are that it is irreversible and can cause severe complications including liver cirrhosis, insulin-dependent diabetes, and hypogonadism [173].

For patients with secondary IOC or severe heart failure, the therapy of choice is chelation agents [185]. Despite poor oral bioavailability and short half-life, deferoxamine treatment is effective at decreasing myocardial iron deposition by approximately 24% and delay onset or reverse early cardiac hemochromatosis [186].

The major challenge in deferoxamine appears to be with long-term compliance [187]. Deferiprone, on the other hand, is an orally active chelation agent used primarily for transfusion-dependent thalassemia patients [165]. Some studies suggest deferiprone is superior to deferoxamine in reducing myocardial iron load [188]. However, current guidelines recommend a combination of the two agents, particularly in patients with heart failure and unstable hemodynamics [189].

Managing patients with signs of heart failure requires a combination of chelation therapy and standard guideline directed heart failure therapy [173]. It is crucial to emphasize that among a cohort of individuals with thalassemia major experiencing heart failure, the amalgamation of routine transfusion-chelation therapy with conventional heart failure treatment yielded a 5-year survival rate similar to a typical heart failure cohort [190]. Certain patients with thalassemia or other hemoglobinopathies may necessitate a gradual up titration and may exhibit a reduced threshold for angiotensin-converting enzyme inhibitors or angiotensin receptor blockers due to decreased arterial blood pressure amid chronic anemia [191]. Lastly, for instances of acute heart failure, intravenous loop diuretics, inotropes, renal replacement therapy, and mechanical circulatory support are employed based on clinical exigencies [191].

9.5 Implications for heart transplantation

While long-term, multicenter data are limited, there is evidence suggesting OHT as a viable therapeutic alternative for patients with cardiac hemochromatosis experiencing severe heart failure refractory to optimal medical treatment and cardiac resynchronization therapy [192]. 10-year survival for patients with cardiac hemochromatosis remains suboptimal at 41% [193]. More recent analysis of the UNOS database found both OHT and combined heart-liver transplantation (CHLT) had 88 and 75% survival at 1- and 2-year intervals, respectively [194]. However, as it stands, patients with hemochromatosis appeared to be much younger with increased waitlist mortality compared to all other etiologies [195]. There has also been a report of CHLT in a patient with hemojuvelin-associated hemochromatosis with acceptable outcomes, further demonstrating the role of solid-organ transplantation in managing cardiac hemochromatosis patients [196]. In patients with persistent congestive heart failure post-liver transplantation, durable or temporary biventricular assist devices may be considered [197]. Most importantly, all patients receiving either OHT or CHLT should continue therapies to decrease the iron load on the transplanted allograft [178].

9.6 Future directions

Abnormalities in hepcidin have been implicated in almost all forms of hereditary hemochromatosis [198]. Recently, phase 2 randomized controlled trial of rusfertide in patients with HFE-related hemochromatosis demonstrated the efficacy of the hepcidin mimetic on preventing re-accumulation of iron without needing phlebotomy [199]. We also await the results from the Thalassemic Iron Overload Cardiomyopathy is Ameliorated by Taurine Supplementation (TICATS) trial [200].

10. Fabry disease

Fabry Disease (FD) is a rare X-linked hereditary lysosomal storage disorder due to pathogenic variants in the *GLA* gene which lead to deficient alpha-galactosidase

A activity. This causes the deposition of toxic globotriaosylceramide (Gb3) in various tissues, including the myocardium [201]. Cardiac involvement manifests with LV hypertrophy, myocardial fibrosis, and arrhythmias, and progresses into heart failure [201]. The advent of enzyme replacement therapy (ERT) has underscored the importance of early detection and intervention to slow disease progression and avert significant cardiac complications [202]. Recent insights into the pathophysiology of FD indicate that, beyond Gb3 buildup, other pathogenic mechanisms contribute to the onset of Fabry cardiomyopathy [203]. Advances in imaging modalities have enhanced the diagnosis and classification of cardiac conditions associated with FD, highlighting the role of myocardial inflammation and paving the way for further investigative endeavors [203]. Furthermore, the rapid evolution of the FD-specific therapeutic landscape, marked by the approval of oral chaperone therapy and novel treatment modalities, signifies promising developments in the field [204].

10.1 Epidemiology

The incidence of FD is estimated to range between 1 in 40,000 to 1 in 170,000 births globally [205]. In Caucasians, incidence can be as high as 1 in 17,000 [205]. In Italy and Japan, newborn males have been screened for FD at rates as high as 1 in 3000, whereas in Taiwan, the rate has been as high as 1 in 1500 [205]. A recent analysis of the United Kingdom Biobank revealed the prevalence of likely pathogenic late-onset variant mutations at 1 in 5732 and the prevalence of mutations causing classic FD at 1 in 200,643 [206]. Notably, later-onset variants were more prevalent in studies focusing on newborn screening, with the ratio of late-onset to classic variants ranging from 7:1 in Italy to 16:1 in Taiwan [207]. These patterns indicate that while mutations related to late-onset FD are more common than mutations associated with classic FD, classic FD is more common in patients with clinically significant FD. Thus, it is plausible that late-onset FD is significantly underdiagnosed [208]. Recent cohort studies on patients with LV hypertrophy indicate a prevalence of FD ranging from 0.3 to 0.9% [209]. Furthermore, the prevalence of FD in unexplained LV hypertrophy is estimated to be even higher, ranging from 2% in Canada to 4% in Hong Kong and the Czech Republic [210].

10.2 Pathophysiology and clinical features

The enzyme alpha-galactosidase normally catalyzes the conversion of Gb3 to lactosylceramide. However, in its deficient or absent state, Gb3 accumulates in the lysosomes, particularly in the cardiovascular endothelium and the nephron, leading to both cardiac and renal abnormalities [211]. The excess infiltration of Gb3 in the myocardium leads to significant oxidative stress, dysfunctional endocytosis, autophagy, and interferes with mitochondrial homeostasis [212]. Beyond the storage cardiomyopathy, diffuse inflammation may play a larger role in FD-driven cardiomyopathy [213]. This in turn provides a valuable target for ERT. The combination of direct infiltration, fibrosis, microvascular ischemia, inflammation, and oxidative stress causes diastolic and systolic dysfunction, leading to symptomatic heart failure. It is estimated that 60% of FD patients develop HFpEF with dyspnea, angina, palpitations, or syncope [10]. Diastolic dysfunction is thought to be more prevalent than systolic dysfunction in FD [214]. However, diastolic dysfunction may manifest with or without LV hypertrophy and play a significant role in the progression of left atrial enlargement and atrial fibrillation [215]. FD is also associated with development of aortic stenosis and regurgitation due to Gb3 deposition within the leaflets or subvalvular apparatus, leading to geometric distortion of the atria, valvular annulus, or aortic root dilation [216].

10.3 Diagnosis

Echocardiography plays a crucial role in the initial identification and continuous monitoring of cardiomyopathy associated with FD [217]. Subtle changes in electrocardiography, such as a shortened PQ interval and aberrations in repolarization, precede the onset of left ventricular hypertrophy (LVH) and can manifest as early as childhood [217]. Over time, individuals may exhibit ST segment depression and T-wave inversion in the inferolateral leads, indicating the development of posterolateral fibrosis. While none are pathognomonic, typical echocardiographic findings include concentric LV hypertrophy, disproportionately large papillary muscles, absence of base-to-apex circumferential strain gradient, and RV hypertrophy with preserved systolic function [218]. Furthermore, CMR provides valuable insights into the myocardial biology of FD at different stages of disease and patients' responsiveness to appropriate therapies. A 3-phase model of cardiac FD progression is as follows: (1) The process of accumulation begins in childhood and is distinguished by a gradual decrease in T1 without LV hypertrophy or LGE. (2) Inflammation and/or hypertrophy manifest with decreased T1 values, initial LV hypertrophy, and T2 mapping indicating inflammation in the basal inferolateral region correlated with LGE. This can sometimes precede LV hypertrophy. (3) Fibrosis and/or functional impairment are characterized by rising T1 values and the presence of LGE along with wall thinning in the basal inferolateral area [219]. In combination with imaging modalities, biomarkers including troponin and NT-proBNP also play an important role in staging cardiac FD [216].

10.4 Management

Enzyme replacement therapy (ERT) is among the first-line treatment of choice for FD and has been shown to be effective in managing neuropathic pain, gastrointestinal symptoms, and heat or exercise tolerance [220]. Long-term observational studies have demonstrated that ERT can delay the progression of cardiac FD, leading to stabilization of LV mass index [221, 222]. Two types of ERTs are currently available: agalsidase-alfa (available in Canada and Europe) and beta (only in the US). A Cochrane review of randomized trial data demonstrates no disparities in cardiac incidents or mortality between patients treated with both formulations [223]. Current guidelines suggest early intervention with ERT, as patients with existing LGE on CMR are less likely to experience regression of LV hypertrophy with ERT. Earlier treatment with ERT has been associated with decreased likelihood of cardiovascular events, including heart failure, arrhythmia, cardiac surgery, LV hypertrophy, atrial fibrillation, and myocardial infarction [224]. However, FD patients with end-stage renal disease or advanced heart failure, characterized by significant myocardial fibrosis, are not expected to benefit from ERT [223]. Immunogenicity of ERT also poses a challenge. Given that ERT is a foreign recombinant protein, patients may develop anti-drug antibodies within 3–6 months of treatment [225]. These responses are thought to be permanent with unknown clinical significance. However, the risk of anti-drug antibody development has been shown to be higher among patients with more severe FD manifestations [226].

Alternatively, chaperone therapy is available for patients who are contraindicated for ERT. Unlike ERT, chaperone therapy is administered orally without risk of immunogenicity. It is important to note that chaperone therapy is only effective in patients with mutations that yield unstable yet functional alpha-galactosidase. However, patients with mutations resulting in deficient enzymes will not respond to chaperone therapy [227]. The efficacy and safety of migalastat has been demonstrated in several trials. The ATTRACT trial, which randomized FD patients to either ERT or transition to migalastat, demonstrated a decrease in LV myocardial index with only migalastat, particularly among those with existing LV hypertrophy [228]. The FACETS trial further corroborated the reduction in LV myocardial index after 2 years among FD patients with baseline LV hypertrophy [202]. More recently, an observational MAIORA study found that the net benefits of migalastat were most pronounced in patients at the initial stages of disease, further underscoring the importance of early treatment [229].

10.5 Implications for heart transplantation

Despite the absence of explicit recommendations, FD is included among the listing criteria for OHT, with the possibility of OHT or combined heart-kidney transplantation (CHKT) at end-stage renal and heart failures [230]. However, outcome data on OHT or CHKT for FD patients is scarce and limited to case reports. A recent report of kidney transplant after OHT has demonstrated excellent outcomes, similar to those seen in CHKT in an FD patient presenting with severe nonobstructive hypertrophic cardiomyopathy and systolic heart failure with reduced EF [231]. Long-term outcomes are also reported to be adequate with one case of an FD patient experiencing recurrence free survival 14 years after OHT [232]. While OHT and CHKT appear to be exceedingly rare for FD patients, they may have significant benefits in patients who have been unresponsive to ERT and chaperone therapy [233]. More data is warranted to better understand the role of solid-organ transplantation among patients with cardiac manifestations of FD.

10.6 Future directions

The MODIFY trial has completed but results are pending regarding the utility of lucerastat oral monotherapy in FD patients [234]. mRNA and gene therapy are another pioneering direction in the treatment of FD. Previously, mRNA therapy has been shown effective in decreasing Gb3 levels in the heart and kidneys in a murine model of FD [235]. When translated into non-human primates, mRNA therapy has been able to augment the alpha-galactosidase activity in the heart, albeit not in the kidneys [236]. As for gene therapy, *GLA* nucleoside-modified messenger RNA (modRNA) treatment has been shown effective in decreasing Gb3 levels in human cardiomyocytes. However, its clinical utility warrants further investigation in human trials [237].

11. Danon disease

Danon disease (DD) is a rare but severe and penetrant form of inherited ICMs. It follows an X-linked inheritance pattern resulting in the deficiency of the lysosomal-associated membrane 2 protein (LAMP-2) [238]. Majority of patients with DD experience severe, symptomatic HFpEF and concurrent neurologic, skeletal, and ophthalmologic complications [239]. Reports of patients with DD cardiomyopathy often denote hearts that are among the largest ever observed [240]. Males tend to be symptomatic at an earlier stage compared to female patients, and most often succumb to heart failure and arrhythmia before 30 years of age or receiving OHT [241].

11.1 Epidemiology

The exact prevalence of DD remains unknown. A study on hypertrophic cardiomyopathy in pediatric patients found that roughly 4% of patients had DD [242]. It has also been observed that roughly 17% of patients with both LV hypertrophy and pre-excitation had DD [242]. However, there are clear gender disparities in the onset of DD, with males presenting earlier with only LV hypertrophy compared to women who present later in the disease process with both LV hypertrophy and dilated cardiomyopathy [243].

11.2 Pathophysiology and clinical features

Severe deficiency in LAMP-2B protein leads to compromised macro-autophagy, leading to accumulation and myocardial infiltration of intracellular vacuoles containing glycogen and other cytoplasmic contents. Dysfunctional autophagy leads to oxidative stress, diffuse fibrosis, and conduction abnormalities [244]. LV hypertrophy is the most common cardiac manifestation for both sexes, likely due to sustained myocardial injury because of impaired autophagy. However, 30–50% of female patients may present with dilated or hypokinetic nondilated cardiomyopathy [243]. Younger patients are more vulnerable to accelerated LV hypertrophy [245]. The hypertrophic heart typically becomes hypokinetic due to cardiomyocyte apoptosis and progressive fibrosis, eventually leading to wall thinning and potentially dilation [246]. Electrophysiological abnormalities and arrhythmias seen in DD cardiomyopathy are highlighted by initial shortening of PR intervals and delta waves, indicating accelerated AV node conduction or the presence of accessory pathways [241]. As the disease progresses, repolarization irregularities and atrial or ventricular arrhythmias develop [247]. It is estimated that 60% of DD patients experience supraventricular tachycardias such as atrial flutter and fibrillation. Pre-excitation associated with Wolff-Parkinson-White syndrome may be an early indicator of DD cardiomyopathy and is more common among males than females. High-degree heart block and sinus node dysfunction is also common, occurring in roughly 35–50% of DD patients [238]. Importantly, patients with DD may initially present with cardiac arrest and sudden fatal arrhythmias [238]. Thus, it is difficult to predict and prevent cardiac manifestations of DD until younger patients present with major adverse cardiac events. Eventually, extensive hypertrophy and conduction disturbances lead to irreversible heart failure [238].

Several extracardiac clinical features merit discussions that may cue clinicians into a diagnosis of DD. Patients may present with proximal muscle weakness and myalgias [248]. Neurocognitive symptoms include learning disabilities and mild cognitive deficits in younger patients. Some may present with unexplained anxiety and mood disorders [243]. Visual manifestations include pigmentary retinopathy and myopia, particularly among male patients [249]. Finally, gastrointestinal manifestations include hepatomegaly and elevated liver enzymes. Patients with advanced heart failure are more likely to experience congestive hepatopathy [241].

11.3 Diagnosis

While definitive diagnosis of DD is dependent on genetic testing for the LAMP2 gene, CMR plays a major role in identifying patterns of hypertrophy and distribution of LGE [1]. In male patients with DD, LV hypertrophy is characterized by concentric patterns of LV wall thickening that may resemble sarcomeric hypertrophic cardiomyopathy [250]. However, EF is often preserved. On the other hand, female DD patients display asymmetric LV, RV hypertrophy or dilated cardiomyopathy [243]. Echocardiograms may also show a high degree of cardiac fibrosis. In combination with Wolff-Parkinson-White syndrome on ECG, this may be an important predictor of future progression of conduction abnormalities [251]. Myocardial biopsy may reveal regular acid maltase levels, thereby distinguishing DD from closely related Pompe disease. Immunohistochemical features include accumulation of autophagic vacuoles and deficient LAMP2 expression [252, 253].

11.4 Management

There are no available medical therapies for DD. It is recommended that the cardiac manifestations of DD should be managed as per appropriate guidelines depending on the phenotype. Often, diuretics, antiarrhythmics, and beta blockers are first-line treatments [241]. It is important to note that since the disease process impairs mitochondrial function, DD patients exhibit low tolerance towards hypertension, tachycardia, and anemia. It is advisable to steer clear of cardiotoxic drugs and stimulants [241]. Recent guidelines suggest that given the progressive fibrosis and systolic dysfunction in DD, therapies such as beta blockers and renin-angiotensin-aldosterone system inhibitors should be considered to attenuate cardiac remodeling [241]. Implantable cardioverter-defibrillators may be considered for patients with moderate to severe cardiomyopathy, especially when they have familial history of premature sudden cardiac death [251].

11.5 Implications for heart transplantation

In the absence of definitive medical therapies for DD, early consideration for OHT is crucial in patients with DD, particularly among young males who carry higher risk of sudden cardiac death and rapid progression of LV hypertrophy [254]. Recent retrospective analysis has shown promising outcomes for DD patients undergoing OHT with a 5-year survival probability of 87.1%, with no significant differences in outcomes between male and female patients [255]. However, large, multicenter data on long-term outcomes are still limited. Post-transplant management should consider the utilization of steroid-sparing immunosuppression to mitigate the risk of further cardiac and skeletal muscle damage [255].

11.6 Future directions

Gene therapy, using viral capsids from adeno-associated viruses (AAV) have been in development for DD [256]. AAV9, for example, has demonstrated enhanced transduction of genetic material in cardiac muscle while minimizing uptake in other tissues. Clinical trials have commenced to assess the effectiveness of AAV9 gene therapy in Danon disease following promising outcomes in mice during preclinical investigations of improved survival and cardiac function post LAMP2B/AAV9 gene therapy

(RP-A501). Initial data from phase 1 clinical trials involving pediatric and adult patients have exhibited positive outcomes, including indications of LAMP2B protein expression, substantial clearance of vacuoles at the tissue level, trends towards decreased levels of troponins and BNP [257]. However, major challenges remain in the medical management of DD. Although gene therapy may alleviate cardiac symptoms, extracardiac manifestations like skeletal myopathy, retinal impairment, and intellectual disability are likely to remain largely unaffected by this intervention [258].

12. Pompe disease

Pompe disease (PD) is a glycogen storage disorder (type 2) inherited in an autosomal recessive pattern leading to pathogenic alterations in the gene encoding acid alpha-glucosidase (GAA). This causes excessive deposition of lysosomal glycogen in cardiac and skeletal muscles [259]. There are two major phenotypes of PD: the classic infantile onset which occurs before 1-year of age with LV hypertrophy or obstruction of the LV outflow tract, and late onset occurring after 1-year of age without hypertrophic cardiomyopathy [260]. Classic infantile PD is aggressive and carries a high mortality rate due to premature heart failure with 75% of patients dying before the age of 1 with median age at death of 8.7 months [260]. Late-onset PD usually do not have cardiac manifestations but may present with muscle weakness and respiratory failure [261]. It is important to recognize that PD is a spectrum with variable organ involvement, onset of symptoms, and degree of cardiomyopathy. Therefore, not all patients may be strictly categorized into the above-mentioned phenotypes [261].

12.1 Epidemiology

PD is estimated to occur in roughly 1 in 40,000 people globally. However, the incidence varies by ethnicity [262]. In the United States, the highest incidence is observed in the African American population, where incidence rates may be as high as 1 in 14,000 [262]. In Europe, it is estimated that incidence of classic infantile onset PD is 1 in 100,000 and late-onset PD occurs in about 1 in 60,000 people [262]. Some studies have identified people of Taiwanese, Dutch, and Israeli descent may be at a higher risk of developing PD [262].

12.2 Pathophysiology and clinical features

In the absence of acid maltase or alpha glucosidase, glycogen accumulates in lysosomal vacuoles and in the cytoplasmic spaces, triggering muscular dysfunction. In addition, toxic lysosomal enzymes may be released due to secondary rupture of lysosomes, further compounding the myocardial breakdown [263]. Similar to DD and other glycogen storage disorders, impaired autophagic function may also play a role in pathogenesis as accumulation of autophagosomes have been reported in PD [264]. In classic infantile-onset PD, right and LV hypertrophy leads to obstruction of the LV outflow tract, abnormal ventricular compliance, and diastolic dysfunction [265]. Infiltrative process of excess glycogen leads to conduction abnormalities which may manifest as elevated QRS voltage, pre-excitation patterns, repolarization anomalies, bundle branch blocks, and AV blocks. Other notable clinical features of classic infantile PD include hypotonia, hepatomegaly, and respiratory insufficiency [266].

In contrast, late-onset PD does not manifest with significant LV hypertrophy despite some evidence of baseline decreases in LV mass and systolic function [267]. Instead, late-onset PD is notable for slowly progressive proximal weakness and more prominent respiratory distress [267, 268].

12.3 Diagnosis

Definitive diagnosis of PD must be made with enzyme assays and genetic testing. Currently, classic infantile-onset PD is screened at birth according to the Recommended Uniform Screening Panel in 29 states as of 2024 [262, 269]. However, assessment of cardiac function by echocardiography is an essential component of PD cardiomyopathy. Initial findings may indicate increased LV wall thickness and mass. This is an important metric as it can be evaluated frequently to establish the stage of cardiomyopathy when determining treatment. Longitudinally, metrics such as 2-dimensional ejection fraction and myocardial performance index are helpful for follow-ups [260]. ECG findings include shortening of the PR interval and commonly Wolf-Parkinson-White syndrome [260]. Therefore, 24-hour ambulatory ECG or Holter monitoring should be considered in patients with suspected PD.

12.4 Management

Akin to FD, ERT is the first-line treatment modality and has been available since 2006. Currently available recombinant human GAA (rhGAA) has shown survival benefits and significant reduction in LV hypertrophy in all PD patients [270]. However, ERT has thus far failed at slowing the progression of disease after childhood. Patients on rhGAA may survive heart or respiratory failures during childhood, but many may experience declines in skeletal muscle strength years after and develop arrhythmias even after LV hypertrophy has been managed. In addition, ERT does not appear to improve other extracardiac features as these patients develop hearing loss, speech issues, cognitive impairments, and gastrointestinal problems as they age [260]. In 2010, a trial with alglucosidase alfa in late-onset PD patients demonstrated some improvements in slowing down motor and respiratory dysfunction. However, these effects only lasted 2–3 years before patients began to return to their gradual decline [271].

More recently, ERT with avalglucosidase alfa (COMET trial) and cipaglucosidase alfa with miglustat (PROPERL trial) has been compared to aglucosidase alfa [272, 273]. Both agents demonstrated non-inferiority to alglucosidase alfa but have not proven any net benefits over the standard of care. While we do not yet have long-term outcomes for these formulations, avalglucosidase alfa and cipaglucosidase alfa with miglustat has been approved for patients with late-onset PD as of 2021 and 2023, respectively [274, 275].

12.5 Implications for heart transplantation

The literature is exceedingly limited regarding OHT for both infantile- and late-onset PD. To our knowledge, there have not been any reports of successful OHT in patients with PD. Late-onset PD patients are likely to be contraindicated for OHT given their significant comorbidities and respiratory complications.

12.6 Future directions

Gene therapy represents the new frontier in treatment for PD. These may be liver-directed or muscle-directed. Currently, we await the results from phase 1/2a trials using one-time intravenous infusion of the AAV-packaged transgene delivered to the liver [276, 277]. This approach will then allow the AAV vectors to create a depot in the liver for GAA production and secretion, even at lower doses of the initial vector infusion. Early preclinical data has demonstrated that these newly produced GAA proteins do not exhibit substantial immunogenicity and have demonstrated significant reduction of glycogen deposition in the cardiac and skeletal muscles [278, 279]. As for the muscle-directed approach, the FORTIS trial is currently underway testing the efficacy of AT845 in adults with late-onset PD [280]. This approach takes advantage of the AAV vector with muscle-specific serotypes and promoters, thereby maximizing the amount of GAA proteins reaching the desired cardiac and skeletal muscle targets [262]. SRT has also been at the forefront of research into PD treatments. Recently, the phase 1 trial of SRT with MZE00, an orally bioavailable inhibitor of glycogen synthase 1, has completed in healthy volunteers. Early results have demonstrated significant reduction of glycogen and phase 2 clinical trial with similar formulation was slated to begin in 2023 [281].

13. Friedreich ataxia

Friedreich ataxia (FRDA), while considered rare, is the most common form of hereditary spinocerebellar ataxia inherited in an autosomal recessive manner [282]. FRDA has a broad spectrum of clinical manifestations, including ataxia of the limbs, trunks, diabetes, and dysarthria. Notably, however, nearly 60% of patients develop cardiomyopathy characterized by LV hypertrophy [283, 284]. The defect or deficiency in the mitochondrial protein frataxin associated with FRDA is thought to be the underlying pathological mechanism of FRDA cardiomyopathy [285]. While the literature is limited on the long-term prognosis and progression, major causes of death among patients with FRDA include sudden cardiac death, congestive heart failure, and arrhythmia [286]. Most patients with FRDA become reliant on wheelchairs within a decade of diagnosis, which further poses challenges for accurately assessing their cardiac function [287]. However, there are several trials on the way that may provide much needed therapeutic interventions for FRDA patients with cardiomyopathy.

13.1 Epidemiology

The global prevalence of FRDA is estimated to be between 1 in 40,000 people, while the carrier frequency appears to be much higher at 1 in 60 to 100 people. FRDA is considered the most common inherited form of ataxia in Europe, the Middle East, Indian subcontinent, and North Africa. However, FRDA has not been documented among other Southeast Asians, sub-Saharan Africans, or among Native Americans [288–290]. In the United States, FRDA is observed in 1 out of 50,000 people, particularly among people of Western European descent. Around 75% of patients with FRDA are under 25 years of age and FRDA does not show any sex disparities [291]. The age of onset is thought to be in early adolescence, often between 8 and 15 years of age [292].

13.2 Pathophysiology and clinical features

Roughly 95% of pathogenesis in FRDA is due to the large triplet expansion in intron 1 of the human FRDA gene, which effectively silences nuclear transcription of the mitochondrial-specific protein frataxin, leading to reduction or deficiency of the protein [285]. This results in iron metabolism dysregulation and mitochondrial dysfunction. Unlike cardiac hemochromatosis, FRDA cardiomyopathy is characterized by the heart's ability to accumulate a significant amount of iron before showing symptoms of heart failure. The reason behind why the limited accumulation of myocardial iron in FRDA is more detrimental than widespread iron overload in hemochromatosis remains unclear [293]. However, FRDA shows an overabundance of ferritin deposition, compared to siderin or hemosiderin seen in cardiac hemochromatosis or IOC [294]. In FRDA, cardiac mitochondria appear in Ferritin deposition, mitochondrial proliferation in the cardiomyocytes, oxidative stress, and localized inflammation leads to moderate to severe LV hypertrophy that is concentric and nonobstructive. This is in stark contrast to sarcomeric cardiomyopathies where defects in sarcomeric contractile proteins lead to obstructive cardiomyopathy and sudden cardiac death [295]. Arrhythmias in FRDA often stem from supraventricular sources, including atrial fibrillation, flutter, and supraventricular tachycardia [286].

13.3 Diagnosis

As with most hereditary causes of ICM, genetic testing is the gold standard for the diagnosis of FRDA. However, imaging and ECG play an important role in understanding the extent of cardiac involvement. ECG generally shows T-wave inversions, left axis deviation, and repolarization abnormalities [296]. Echocardiography is a critical tool in diagnosis of FRDA and several features have been associated with poor prognosis. Notably, LVEF and LV mass may have mutually exclusive predictive values [287]. Importantly, echocardiography is predictive of outcomes in FRDA-associated heart failure only if the LV ejection fraction is below 40% [297, 298]. This is an important distinction to consider in clinical trials as it may help delineate clinically significant predictors of heart failure in FRDA apart from overt progression of disease. CMR is also an important modality to consider. T1 mapping and LGE may demonstrate an increase in extracellular volume and cardiomyocyte size, both of which are linked to more severe cardiomyopathy [299]. T2 imaging may also be useful in quantifying the ventricular size, mass, and myocardial iron load [1]. CMR can detect fibrosis and can provide useful insights regarding the myocardial fiber size, which may be associated with long-term prognosis and aid in risk stratification for FRDA [300]. The role of the right ventricular function warrants further investigation and discussion. A recent study demonstrated that the peak velocities in the RV were lower in patients with FRDA without heart failure, indicating some early impairments in the long-axis function [301]. However, RV remains difficult to image by transthoracic echocardiography. Thus, when examining the RV function, CMR may provide better insights into the RV function.

13.4 Management

There is no treatment of choice for FRDA cardiomyopathy and management strategies remain limited to heart failure medications, antiarrhythmics, and mechanical circulatory support devices in severe cases [10].

13.5 Implications for heart transplantation

In the absence of effective medical management for FRDA cardiomyopathy, OHT may provide treatment with curative intent, especially among patients with end-stage congestive heart failure due to severe LV hypertrophy, fibrosis, and eventual ventricular thinning [302]. In a case series, OHT demonstrated adequate long-term outcomes in patients with severe end-stage heart failure. Importantly, the 22-year follow-up showed that survival in FRDA after OHT was determined by the degree of cardiac involvement and patients with progressive decline in LVEF had worse prognosis after OHT [302]. A more recent case report also demonstrated that patients with advanced FRDA may benefit from OHT, despite the need for higher doses of vasopressors, hemofiltration and delayed tracheal extubation [303]. Whether FRDA should be a contraindication for OHT remains unclear with limited evidence in the literature. However, an important concept to consider is the fact that life expectancy due to FRDA exceeds the median graft survival time, OHT may be a viable treatment option for cardiomyopathy for select patients [303]. Furthermore, there are critical ethical considerations when evaluating potential transplant recipients with progressive neurological disease. This requires a multidisciplinary team to evaluate a wide variety of factors [304].

13.6 Future directions

Intravenous delivery of AAV-vector expressing frataxin has shown some promising results in a murine model of FRDA in its ability to stop the onset or reverse existing heart failure [305]. There have also been studies involving anti-IL6 or anti-IL6 receptor therapies to reduce overt inflammation in FRDA [306]. However, human trials on these strategies have not been conducted. Currently, there are several clinical trials regarding therapeutics for FRDA. Notably, a study with rhAAV transfer vector coding for the frataxin gene is underway with the hope of analyzing its effects on cardiopulmonary function [307]. RT0001, designed to reduce lipid peroxidation from oxidative stress in the mitochondrial membrane, has recently completed recruitment and we await its results on the cardiopulmonary functions of patients with FRDA [308].

14. Conclusions

ICMs encompass a diverse group of myocardial diseases characterized by unique infiltrative pathologies that culminate in restrictive cardiac dysfunction, progressive heart failure, and significant morbidity and mortality. Heart transplantation emerges as a critical therapeutic consideration, particularly for patient's refractory to standard medical interventions. While orthotopic heart transplantation presents as a viable, curative intent for conditions such as cardiac amyloidosis, sarcoidosis, and hemochromatosis, the complexity inherent in each disease process necessitates careful patient selection and individualized pre- and post-transplant management strategies. In amyloidosis, concurrent autologous stem cell transplantation or targeted therapies can significantly enhance post-transplant outcomes, underscoring the importance of a multidisciplinary approach to management. Similarly, heart transplantation outcomes in cardiac sarcoidosis patients parallel those with other cardiomyopathies, although the presence of extracardiac involvement and immunosuppressive complications demands heightened vigilance.

Furthermore, advances in diagnostic modalities, such as cardiac magnetic resonance imaging and biomarker analyses, enhance the early identification of transplant candidates and facilitate risk stratification. Emerging therapeutic innovations, including gene therapy, enzyme replacement, immunotherapies, and RNA silencers, indicate promising future directions in treating infiltrative diseases, potentially altering transplantation paradigms. Despite these advances, significant challenges remain, particularly in managing disease recurrence, balancing immunosuppression, and addressing systemic complications. Continued research and collaboration across disciplines will be vital in refining transplant criteria, optimizing patient outcomes, and advancing therapeutic strategies in ICMs.

Acknowledgements

We thank the Pauley Heart Center for excellent research support and clinical guidance for this work.

Conflict of interest

The authors declare no conflict of interest.

Author details

Ye In Christopher Kwon[1*], Eleanor E. Bashian[2], Elizabeth J. Bashian[1], Justin Chang[3], Valentina Robila[3], Keyur B. Shah[4], Mohammed Makkiya[4] and Zubair A. Hashmi[1]

1 Division of Cardiothoracic Surgery, Department of Surgery, Pauley Heart Center, Virginia Commonwealth University School of Medicine, Richmond, VA, USA

2 Department of Molecular Medicine, The Scripps Research Institute, San Diego, CA, USA

3 Department of Pathology, Virginia Commonwealth University School of medicine, Richmond, VA, USA

4 Division of Cardiology, Department of Internal Medicine, Pauley Heart Center, Virginia Commonwealth University School of Medicine, Richmond, VA, USA

*Address all correspondence to: kwonyc@vcu.edu

References

[1] Kottam A et al. State-of-the-art imaging of infiltrative cardiomyopathies: A scientific statement from the American heart association. Circulation. Cardiovascular Imaging. 2023;**16**(11):e000081

[2] Albakri A. Infiltrative cardiomyopathy: A review of literature on clinical status and meta-analysis of diagnostic and clinical management methods. Clinical and Medical Investigations. 2018;**3**(2). DOI: 10.15761/CMI.1000160

[3] Shah KB, Inoue Y, Mehra MR. Amyloidosis and the heart: A comprehensive review. Archives of Internal Medicine. 2006;**166**(17):1805-1813

[4] Sekhri V, Sanal S, Delorenzo LJ, Aronow WS, Maguire GP. Cardiac sarcoidosis: A comprehensive review. Archives of Medical Science. 2011;7(4):546-554

[5] Sweet ME, Mestroni L, Taylor MRG. Genetic infiltrative cardiomyopathies. Heart Failure Clinics. 2018;**14**(2):215-224

[6] Bengel FM, Ross TL. Emerging imaging targets for infiltrative cardiomyopathy: Inflammation and fibrosis. Journal of Nuclear Cardiology. 2019;**26**(1):208-216

[7] Rimoldi O, Maranta F. Microvascular dysfunction in infiltrative cardiomyopathies. Journal of Nuclear Cardiology. 2019;**26**(1):200-207

[8] Wechalekar AD, Gillmore JD, Hawkins PN. Systemic amyloidosis. Lancet. 2016;**387**(10038):2641-2654

[9] Kittleson MM, Maurer MS, Ambardekar AV. Cardiac amyloidosis: Evolving diagnosis and management: A scientific statement from the American Heart Association [published correction appears in circulation]. Circulation. 2021;**144**(1):e10. DOI: 10.1161/CIR.0000000000000997

[10] Bejar D, Colombo PC, Latif F, Yuzefpolskaya M. Infiltrative cardiomyopathies. Clinical Medicine Insights: Cardiology. 2015;**9**(Suppl. 2):19706. DOI: 10.4137/CMC.S19706

[11] Varga C et al. The diagnostic challenges of cardiac amyloidosis: A practical approach to the two main types. Blood Reviews. 2021;**45**:100720

[12] Ruberg FL, Grogan M, Hanna M, Kelly JW, Maurer MS. Transthyretin amyloid cardiomyopathy: JACC state-of-the-art review. Journal of the American College of Cardiology. 2019;**73**(22):2872-2891

[13] Falk RH, Alexander KM, Liao R, Dorbala S. AL (light-chain) cardiac amyloidosis: A review of diagnosis and therapy. Journal of the American College of Cardiology. 2016;**68**(12):1323-1341. DOI: 10.1016/j.jacc.2016.06.053

[14] Kyle RA et al. Incidence of AL amyloidosis in Olmsted County, Minnesota, 1990 through 2015. Mayo Clinic Proceedings. 2019;**94**(3):465-471

[15] Wan H, Goodkind D, Kowal P. US Census Bureau, International Population Reports, P95/16-1, An Aging World: 2015. US Government Publishing Office; 2016 [Online]. Available from: https://www.census.gov/content/dam/Census/library/publications/2016/demo/p95-16-1.pdf

[16] Gilstrap LG et al. Epidemiology of cardiac amyloidosis-associated heart

failure hospitalizations among fee-for-service Medicare beneficiaries in the United States. Circulation. Heart Failure. 2019;**12**(6):e005407

[17] Merlini G, Bellotti V. Molecular mechanisms of amyloidosis. The New England Journal of Medicine. 2003;**349**(6):583-596

[18] Kushwaha SS, Fallon JT, Fuster V. Restrictive cardiomyopathy. The New England Journal of Medicine. 1997;**336**(4):267-276

[19] Roberts WC, Waller BF. Cardiac amyloidosis causing cardiac dysfunction: Analysis of 54 necropsy patients. The American Journal of Cardiology. 1983;**52**(1):137-146

[20] Ridolfi RL, Bulkley BH, Hutchins GM. The conduction system in cardiac amyloidosis. Clinical and pathologic features of 23 patients. The American Journal of Medicine. 1977;**62**(5):677-686

[21] Smith RR, Hutchins GM. Ischemic heart disease secondary to amyloidosis of intramyocardial arteries. The American Journal of Cardiology. 1979;**44**(3):413-417

[22] Neben-Wittich MA, Wittich CM, Mueller PS, Larson DR, Gertz MA, Edwards WD. Obstructive intramural coronary amyloidosis and myocardial ischemia are common in primary amyloidosis. The American Journal of Medicine. 2005;**118**(11):1287

[23] Wu D, Chen W. Molecular mechanisms and emerging therapies in wild-type transthyretin amyloid cardiomyopathy. Heart Failure Reviews. 2024;**29**(2):511-521

[24] Falk RH, Dubrey SW. Amyloid heart disease. Progress in Cardiovascular Diseases. 2010;**52**(4):347-361

[25] Kraemer BF, Seizer P, Geisler T. Persistent troponin elevation in a patient with cardiac amyloidosis. Clinical Cardiology. 2009;**32**(11)

[26] Cantwell RV, Aviles RJ, Bjornsson J. Cardiac amyloidosis presenting with elevations of cardiac troponin I and angina pectoris. Clinical Cardiology. 2002;**25**(1):33-37

[27] Chamarthi B, Dubrey SW, Cha K, Skinner M, Falk RH. Features and prognosis of exertional syncope in light-chain associated AL cardiac amyloidosis. The American Journal of Cardiology. 1997;**80**(9):1242-1245

[28] Mathew V, Olson LJ, Gertz MA, Hayes DL. Symptomatic conduction system disease in cardiac amyloidosis. The American Journal of Cardiology. 1997;**80**(11):1491-1492

[29] Navarro JF, Rivera M, Ortuno J. Cardiac tamponade as presentation of systemic amyloidosis. International Journal of Cardiology. 1992;**36**(1):107-108

[30] Feng D, Edwards WD, Oh JK. Intracardiac thrombosis and embolism in patients with cardiac amyloidosis. Circulation. 2007;**116**(21):2420-2426

[31] Perfetti V et al. The repertoire of λ light chains causing predominant amyloid heart involvement and identification of a preferentially involved germline gene, IGLV1-44. Blood. 2012;**119**(1):144-150

[32] Stelmach-Gołdyś A et al. Physiology, diagnosis and treatment of cardiac light chain amyloidosis. Journal of Clinical Medicine. 2022;**11**(4):911

[33] Marin-Argany M et al. Cell damage in light chain amyloidosis. Journal of Biological Chemistry.

2016;**291**(38):19813-19825. DOI: 10.1074/jbc.M116.736736

[34] Merlini G. AL amyloidosis: From molecular mechanisms to targeted therapies. Hematology. American Society of Hematology. Education Program. 2017;**2017**(1):1-12

[35] Maleszewski JJ. Cardiac amyloidosis: Pathology, nomenclature, and typing. Cardiovascular Pathology. 2015;**24**(6):343-350

[36] Esplin BL, Gertz MA. Current trends in diagnosis and Management of Cardiac Amyloidosis. Current Problems in Cardiology. 2013;**38**(2):53-96. DOI: 10.1016/j.cpcardiol.2012.11.002

[37] Kumar S et al. Revised prognostic staging system for light chain amyloidosis incorporating cardiac biomarkers and serum free light chain measurements. Journal of Clinical Oncology. 2012;**30**(9):989-995

[38] Berk JL et al. Persistent pleural effusions in primary systemic amyloidosis. Chest. 2003;**124**(3):969-977. DOI: 10.1378/chest.124.3.969

[39] Ruberg FL, Berk JL. Transthyretin (TTR) cardiac amyloidosis. Circulation. 2012;**126**(10):1286-1300

[40] Quarta CC et al. The amyloidogenic V122I transthyretin variant in elderly black Americans. The New England Journal of Medicine. 2015;**372**(1):21-29. DOI: 10.1056/NEJMoa1404852

[41] Castaño A, Drachman BM, Judge D, Maurer MS. Natural history and therapy of TTR-cardiac amyloidosis: Emerging disease-modifying therapies from organ transplantation to stabilizer and silencer drugs. Heart Failure Reviews. 2015;**20**(2):163-178. DOI: 10.1007/S10741-014-9462-7/FIGURES/2

[42] Connors LH et al. Heart failure resulting from age-related cardiac amyloid disease associated with wild-type transthyretin: A prospective, observational cohort study. Circulation. 2016;**133**(3):282-290

[43] Hahn VS et al. Endomyocardial biopsy characterization of heart failure with preserved ejection fraction and prevalence of cardiac amyloidosis. JACC. Heart Failure. 2020;**8**(9):712-724. DOI: 10.1016/j.jchf.2020.04.007

[44] González-López E et al. Wild-type transthyretin amyloidosis as a cause of heart failure with preserved ejection fraction. European Heart Journal. 2015;**36**(38):2585-2594. DOI: 10.1093/eurheartj/ehv338

[45] Donnellan E et al. Atrial fibrillation in transthyretin cardiac amyloidosis: Predictors, prevalence, and efficacy of rhythm control strategies. JACC. Clinical Electrophysiology. 2020;**6**(9):1118-1127

[46] Khanna S, Lo P, Cho K, Subbiah R. Ventricular arrhythmias in cardiac amyloidosis: A review of current literature. Clinical Medicine Insights. Cardiology. 2020;**14**:1179546820963055

[47] Godara A et al. Association between spinal stenosis and wild-type ATTR amyloidosis. Amyloid. 2021;**28**(4):226-233. DOI: 10.1080/13506129.2021.1950681

[48] Maurer MS et al. Analysis of lumbar spine stenosis specimens for identification of amyloid. Journal of the American Geriatrics Society. 2022;**70**(12):3538-3548. DOI: 10.1111/jgs.17976

[49] Jacobson DR, Buxbaum JN. Genetic aspects of amyloidosis. Advances in Human Genetics. 1991;**2069**:123

[50] Liu PP, Smyth D. Wild-type transthyretin amyloid cardiomyopathy:

A missed cause of heart failure with preserved ejection fraction with evolving treatment implications. Circulation. 2016;**133**(3):245-247

[51] Pitkänen CGP 3rd, Westermark P. Senile systemic amyloidosis. The American Journal of Pathology. 1984;**117**(3):391-399

[52] Buxbaum JN, Tagoe C, Gallo G, Walker JR, Kurian S, Salomon DR. Why are some amyloidoses systemic? Does hepatic "chaperoning at a distance" prevent cardiac deposition in a transgenic model of human senile systemic (transthyretin) amyloidosis? The FASEB Journal. 2012;**26**(6):2283-2293. DOI: 10.1096/fj.11-189571

[53] Tanskanen M et al. Senile systemic amyloidosis affects 25% of the very aged and associates with genetic variation in alpha2-macroglobulin and tau: A population-based autopsy study. Annals of Medicine. 2008;**40**(3):232-239. DOI: 10.1080/07853890701842988

[54] Brailovsky Y, Rajapreyar I, Alvarez R. TTR amyloidosis: Current state of affairs and promise for the future. JACC. Case Reports. 2023;**10**:101759

[55] Westin O et al. Screening for cardiac amyloidosis 5 to 15 years after surgery for bilateral carpal tunnel syndrome. Journal of the American College of Cardiology. 2022;**80**(10):967-977. DOI: 10.1016/j.jacc.2022.06.026

[56] Dubrey SW, Cha K, Simms RW, Skinner M, Falk RH. Electrocardiography and Doppler echocardiography in secondary (AA) amyloidosis. The American Journal of Cardiology. 1996;77(4):313-315

[57] Gillmore JD, Lovat LB, Persey MR, Pepys MB, Hawkins PN. Amyloid load and clinical outcome in AA amyloidosis in relation to circulating concentration of serum amyloid a protein. Lancet. 2001;**358**(9275):24-29

[58] Westermark P, Johansson B, Natvig JB. Senile cardiac amyloidosis: Evidence of two different amyloid substances in the ageing heart. Scandinavian Journal of Immunology. 1979;**10**:303-308

[59] Kawamura S, Takahashi M, Ishihara T, Uchino F. Incidence and distribution of isolated atrial amyloid: Histologic and immunohistochemical studies of 100 aging hearts. Pathology International. 1995;**45**:335-342

[60] Looi LM. Isolated atrial amyloidosis: A clinicopathologic study indicating increased prevalence in chronic heart disease. Human Pathology. 1993;**24**:602-607

[61] Röcken C et al. Atrial amyloidosis: An arrhythmogenic substrate for persistent atrial fibrillation. Circulation. 2002;**106**(16):2091-2097. DOI: 10.1161/01.cir.0000034511.06350.df

[62] Leone O et al. Amyloid deposition as a cause of atrial remodelling in persistent valvular atrial fibrillation. European Heart Journal. 2004;**25**(14):1237-1241. DOI: 10.1016/j.ehj.2004.04.007

[63] Maceira AM et al. Cardiovascular magnetic resonance in cardiac amyloidosis. Circulation. 2005;**111**(2):186-193

[64] Dorbala S et al. ASNC/AHA/ASE/EANM/HFSA/ISA/SCMR/SNMMI expert consensus recommendations for multimodality imaging in cardiac amyloidosis: Part 1 of 2-evidence base and standardized methods of imaging. Circulation. Cardiovascular Imaging. 2021;**14**(7):e000029

[65] Singh V, Dorbala S. Positron emission tomography for cardiac amyloidosis: Timing matters! Journal of Nuclear Cardiology. 2022;**29**(2):790-797

[66] Davies DR et al. A simple score to identify increased risk of transthyretin amyloid cardiomyopathy in heart failure with preserved ejection fraction. JAMA Cardiology. 2022;**7**(10):1036-1044

[67] Ribeiro Neto ML et al. Performance of diagnostic criteria in patients clinically judged to have cardiac sarcoidosis: Is it time to regroup? American Heart Journal. 2020;**223**:106-109

[68] Kastritis E et al. Daratumumab-based treatment for immunoglobulin light-chain amyloidosis. New England Journal of Medicine. 2021;**385**(1):46-58. DOI: 10.1056/NEJMOA2028631/SUPPL_FILE/NEJMOA2028631_DATA-SHARING.PDF

[69] Shen KN et al. Doxycycline combined with Bortezomib-cyclophosphamide-dexamethasone chemotherapy for newly diagnosed cardiac light-chain amyloidosis: A Multicenter randomized controlled trial. Circulation. 2022;**145**(1):8-17. DOI: 10.1161/CIRCULATIONAHA.121.055953

[70] Palladini G, Milani P, Merlini G. Management of AL amyloidosis in 2020. Blood. 2020;**136**(23):2620-2627. DOI: 10.1182/BLOOD.2020006913

[71] Kittleson MM et al. ACC expert consensus decision pathway on comprehensive multidisciplinary Care for the Patient with Cardiac Amyloidosis. Journal of the American College of Cardiology. 2023;**81**(11):1076-1126. DOI: 10.1016/j.jacc.2022.11.022

[72] Maurer MS et al. Patisiran treatment in patients with transthyretin cardiac amyloidosis. New England Journal of Medicine. 2023;**389**(17):1553-1565. DOI: 10.1056/NEJMoa2300757

[73] Maurer MS et al. Tafamidis treatment for patients with transthyretin amyloid cardiomyopathy. New England Journal of Medicine. 2018;**379**(11):1007-1016. DOI: 10.1056/NEJMOA1805689/SUPPL_FILE/NEJMOA1805689_DATA-SHARING.PDF

[74] Ibrahim M et al. The use of diflunisal for transthyretin cardiac amyloidosis: A review. Heart Failure Reviews. 2022;**27**(2):517-524. DOI: 10.1007/s10741-021-10143-4

[75] Dey BR, Chung SS, Spitzer TR, Zheng H, Macgillivray TE, Seldin DC. Cardiac transplantation followed by dose-intensive melphalan and autologous stem-cell transplantation for light chain amyloidosis and heart failure. Transplantation. 2010;**90**(8):905-911

[76] Lacy MQ, Dispenzieri A, Hayman SR, et al. Autologous stem cell transplant after heart transplant for light chain (Al) amyloid cardiomyopathy. The Journal of Heart and Lung Transplantation. 2008;**27**(8):823-829. DOI: 10.1016/j.healun.2008.05.016

[77] Varr BC, Liedtke M, Arai S, Lafayette RA, Schrier SL, Witteles RM. Heart transplantation and cardiac amyloidosis: Approach to screening and novel management strategies. The Journal of Heart and Lung Transplantation. 2012;**31**(3):325-331

[78] Estep JD, Bhimaraj A, Cordero-Reyes AM, Bruckner B, Loebe M, Torre-Amione G. Heart transplantation and end-stage cardiac amyloidosis: A review and approach to evaluation and management. Methodist DeBakey Cardiovascular Journal. 2012;**8**(3):8-16

[79] Dubrey SW, Burke MM, Hawkins PN, Banner NR. Cardiac transplantation for amyloid heart disease: The United Kingdom experience. The Journal of Heart and Lung Transplantation. 2004;**23**(10):1142-1153

[80] Pelosi F Jr, Capehart J, Roberts WC. Effectiveness of cardiac transplantation for primary (AL) cardiac amyloidosis. The American Journal of Cardiology. 1997;**79**(4):532-535

[81] Johnson MR, Meyer KH, Haft J, Kinder D, Webber SA, Dyke DB. Heart transplantation in the United States, 1999-2008. American Journal of Transplantation. 2010;**10**(4 Pt 2):1035-1046. DOI: 10.1111/j.1600-6143.2010.03042.x

[82] Barrett CD et al. Outcomes in patients with cardiac amyloidosis undergoing heart transplantation. JACC. Heart Failure. 2020;**8**(6):461-468

[83] Witteles RM. Cardiac transplantation and mechanical circulatory support in amyloidosis. JACC. CardioOncology. 2021;**3**(4):516-521

[84] Maurer MS et al. Cardiac transplantation using extended-donor criteria organs for systemic amyloidosis complicated by heart failure. Transplantation. 2007;**83**(5):539-545. DOI: 10.1097/01.tp.0000255567.80203.bd

[85] Gray Gilstrap L et al. Predictors of survival to orthotopic heart transplant in patients with light chain amyloidosis. The Journal of Heart and Lung Transplantation. 2014;**33**(2):149-156. DOI: 10.1016/j.healun.2013.09.004

[86] O. Procurement and T. Network. US Department of Health and Human Services. Criteria Requirements in Adult Heart Allocation Policy. [Online]. Available from: https://optn.transplant.hrsa.gov/media/2413/adult_heart_criteria.pdf

[87] Griffin JM et al. United network for organ sharing outcomes after heart transplantation for al compared to ATTR cardiac amyloidosis. Clinical Transplantation. 2020;**34**(10):e14028. DOI: 10.1111/ctr.14028

[88] Gertz MA et al. First-in-human phase I/II study of NEOD001 in patients with light chain amyloidosis and persistent organ dysfunction. Journal of Clinical Oncology. 2016;**34**(10):1097-1103. DOI: 10.1200/JCO.2015.63.6530

[89] Ward JE et al. Doxycycline reduces fibril formation in a transgenic mouse model of AL amyloidosis. Blood. 2011;**118**(25):6610-6617. DOI: 10.1182/BLOOD-2011-04-351643

[90] Biolo A et al. Matrix metalloproteinases and their tissue inhibitors in cardiac amyloidosis: Relationship to structural, functional myocardial changes and to light chain amyloid deposition. Circulation. Heart Failure. 2008;**1**(4):249-257. DOI: 10.1161/CIRCHEARTFAILURE.108.788687

[91] Wechalekar AD, Whelan C. Encouraging impact of doxycycline on early mortality in cardiac light chain (AL) amyloidosis. Blood Cancer Journal. 2017;7(3):546-546. DOI: 10.1038/bcj.2017.26

[92] Gertz MA et al. Birtamimab plus standard of care in light-chain amyloidosis: The phase 3 randomized placebo-controlled VITAL trial. Blood. 2023;**142**(14):1208-1218. DOI: 10.1182/BLOOD.2022019406/2060254/BLOOD.2022019406.PDF

[93] P. Corporation. Prothena Announces Confirmatory Phase 3 AFFIRM-AL Study of Birtamimab in Mayo Stage IV

Patients with AL Amyloidosis under SPA Agreement with FDA. 2021

[94] Wechalekar A, Palladini G, Molina MA. PB2150: Cardiac amyloid reaching for extended survival (cares) trials: 2 placebo-controlled, double-blind, randomized, phase 3 trials assessing cael-101 in patients with mayo stages IIIA/IIIB AL amyloidosis. Hema. 2023;**7**(Suppl.). DOI: 10.1097/01.HS9.0000975360.99077.6f

[95] Adams D, Tournev IL, Taylor MS, et al. Efficacy and safety of vutrisiran for patients with hereditary transthyretin-mediated amyloidosis with polyneuropathy: A randomized clinical trial. Amyloid. 2023;**30**(1):1-9. DOI: 10.1080/13506129.2022.2091985

[96] Adams D et al. Patisiran, an RNAi therapeutic, for hereditary transthyretin amyloidosis. The New England Journal of Medicine. 2018;**379**(1):11-21. DOI: 10.1056/NEJMoa1716153

[97] Benson MD, Waddington-Cruz M, Berk JL, et al. Inotersen treatment for patients with hereditary transthyretin amyloidosis. The New England Journal of Medicine. 2018;**379**(1):22-31. DOI: 10.1056/NEJMoa1716793

[98] Griffin JM, Rosenthal JL, Grodin JL, Maurer MS, Grogan M, Cheng RK. ATTR amyloidosis: Current and emerging management strategies: JACC: CardioOncology state-of-the-art review. JACC. CardioOncology. 2021;**3**(4):488-505. DOI: 10.1016/j.jaccao.2021.06.006

[99] A Study of PRX004 in Subjects with Amyloid Transthyretin (ATTR) Amyloidosis. ClinicalTrials.gov [Online]. Available from: https://clinicaltrials.gov/ct2/show/NCT03336580?term=NCT03336580&draw=2&rank=1

[100] Gillmore JD et al. CRISPR-Cas9 In vivo gene editing for transthyretin amyloidosis. The New England Journal of Medicine. 2021;**385**(6):493-502. DOI: 10.1056/NEJMoa2107454

[101] Birnie DH, Nery PB, Ha AC, Beanlands RSB. Cardiac sarcoidosis. Journal of the American College of Cardiology. 2016;**68**(4):411-421

[102] McGrath DS, Goh N, Foley PJ, Bois RM. Sarcoidosis: Genes and microbes–soil or seed? Sarcoidosis, Vasculitis, and Diffuse Lung Diseases. 2001;**18**(2):149-164

[103] Valeyre D, Prasse A, Nunes H, Uzunhan Y, Brillet PY, Müller-Quernheim J. Sarcoidosis. Lancet. 2014;**383**(9923):1155-1167. DOI: 10.1016/S0140-6736(13)60680-7

[104] Morimoto T et al. Epidemiology of sarcoidosis in Japan. The European Respiratory Journal. 2008;**31**(2):372-379

[105] Hillerdal G, Nöu E, Osterman K, Schmekel B. Sarcoidosis: Epidemiology and prognosis. A 15-year European study. The American Review of Respiratory Disease. 1984;**130**(1):29-32. DOI: 10.1164/arrd.1984.130.1.29

[106] Rybicki BA, Iannuzzi MC, Frederick MM. Familial aggregation of sarcoidosis. A case-control etiologic study of sarcoidosis (ACCESS). American Journal of Respiratory and Critical Care Medicine. 2001;**164**(11):2085-2091. DOI: 10.1164/ajrccm.164.11.2106001

[107] Iwai K, Tachibana T, Takemura T, Matsui Y, Kitaichi M, Kawabata Y. Pathological studies on sarcoidosis autopsy. I. Epidemiological features of 320 cases in Japan. Acta Pathologica Japonica. 1993;**43**(7):372-376. DOI: 10.1111/j.1440-1827.1993.tb01148.x

[108] Perry A, Vuitch F. Causes of death in patients with sarcoidosis. A

morphologic study of 38 autopsies with clinicopathologic correlations. Archives of Pathology & Laboratory Medicine. 1995;**119**(2):167-172

[109] Murtagh G, Laffin LJ, Beshai JF. Prognosis of myocardial damage in sarcoidosis patients with preserved left ventricular ejection fraction: Risk stratification using cardiovascular magnetic resonance. Circulation. Cardiovascular Imaging. 2016;**9**(1). DOI: 10.1161/CIRCIMAGING.115.003738

[110] Kandolin R, Lehtonen J, Airaksinen J. Cardiac sarcoidosis: Epidemiology, characteristics, and outcome over 25 years in a nationwide study. Circulation. 2015;**131**(7):624-632. DOI: 10.1161/CIRCULATIONAHA.114.011522

[111] Al-Kindi SG, Oliveira GH. Letter by Al-Kindi and Oliveira regarding article 'cardiac sarcoidosis: Epidemiology, characteristics, and outcome over 25 years in a nationwide study. Circulation. 2015;**132**(17). DOI: 10.1161/CIRCULATIONAHA.115.016258

[112] Arkema EV, Cozier YC. Sarcoidosis epidemiology: Recent estimates of incidence, prevalence and risk factors. Current Opinion in Pulmonary Medicine. 2020;**26**(5):527-534. DOI: 10.1097/MCP.0000000000000715

[113] Birnie DH, Sauer WH, Bogun F. HRS expert consensus statement on the diagnosis and management of arrhythmias associated with cardiac sarcoidosis. Heart Rhythm. 2014;**11**(7):1305-1323. DOI: 10.1016/j.hrthm.2014.03.043

[114] Baughman RP, Field S, Costabel U. Sarcoidosis in America. Analysis based on health care use. Annals of the American Thoracic Society. 2016;**13**(8):1244-1252. DOI: 10.1513/AnnalsATS.201511-760OC

[115] Cozier YC, Berman JS, Palmer JR, Boggs DA, Serlin DM, Rosenberg L. Sarcoidosis in black women in the United States: Data from the black Women's Health Study. Chest. 2011;**139**(1):144-150. DOI: 10.1378/chest.10-0413

[116] Mirsaeidi M, Machado RF, Schraufnagel D, Sweiss NJ, Baughman RP. Racial difference in sarcoidosis mortality in the United States. Chest. 2015;**147**(2):438-449. DOI: 10.1378/chest.14-1120

[117] Mathai SV, Patel S, Jorde UP, Epidemiology RY. Pathogenesis, and diagnosis of cardiac sarcoidosis. Methodist DeBakey Cardiovascular Journal. 2022;**18**(2):78-93. DOI: 10.14797/mdcvj.1057

[118] Kandolin R, Lehtonen J, Kupari M. Cardiac sarcoidosis and giant cell myocarditis as causes of atrioventricular block in young and middle-aged adults. Circulation. Arrhythmia and Electrophysiology. 2011;**4**(3):303-309. DOI: 10.1161/CIRCEP.110.959254

[119] Nery PB, Beanlands RS, Nair GM. Atrioventricular block as the initial manifestation of cardiac sarcoidosis in middle-aged adults. Journal of Cardiovascular Electrophysiology. 2014;**25**(8):875-881. DOI: 10.1111/jce.12401

[120] Segura AM, Radovancevic R, Demirozu ZT, Frazier OH, Buja LM. Granulomatous myocarditis in severe heart failure patients undergoing implantation of a left ventricular assist device. Cardiovascular Pathology. 2014;**23**(1):17-20. DOI: 10.1016/j.carpath.2013.06.005

[121] Naruse TK, Matsuzawa Y, Ota M. HLA-DQB1*0601 is primarily associated with the susceptibility to cardiac sarcoidosis. Tissue

Antigens. 2000;**56**(1):52-57. DOI: 10.1034/j.1399-0039.2000.560107.x

[122] Takashige N, Naruse TK, Matsumori A. Genetic polymorphisms at the tumour necrosis factor loci (TNFA and TNFB) in cardiac sarcoidosis. Tissue Antigens. 1999;**54**(2):191-193. DOI: 10.1034/j.1399-0039.1999.540211.x

[123] Berlin M, Fogdell-Hahn A, Olerup O, Eklund A, Grunewald J. HLA-DR predicts the prognosis in Scandinavian patients with pulmonary sarcoidosis. American Journal of Respiratory and Critical Care Medicine. 1997;**156**(5):1601-1605. DOI: 10.1164/ajrccm.156.5.9704069

[124] Ezzie ME, Crouser ED. Considering an infectious etiology of sarcoidosis. Clinics in Dermatology. 2007;**25**(3):259-266. DOI: 10.1016/j.clindermatol.2007.03.003

[125] Giblin GT et al. Cardiac sarcoidosis: When and how to treat inflammation. Cardiac Failure Review. 2021;7. DOI: 10.15420/CFR.2021.16

[126] Lagana SM, Parwani AV, Nichols LC. Cardiac sarcoidosis: A pathology-focused review. Archives of Pathology & Laboratory Medicine. 2010;**134**(7):1039-1046. DOI: 10.5858/2009-0274-RA.1

[127] Liu Y, Qiu L, Wang Y. The circulating Treg/Th17 cell ratio is correlated with relapse and treatment response in pulmonary sarcoidosis patients after corticosteroid withdrawal. PLoS One. 2016;**11**(2):e0148207. DOI: 10.1371/journal.pone.0148207

[128] Gilotra NA et al. "Sarcoidosis-related cardiomyopathy: Current knowledge," challenges, and future perspectives state-of-the-art review. Journal of Cardiac Failure. 2022;**28**(1):113-132. DOI: 10.1016/J.CARDFAIL.2021.06.016

[129] Ramstein J, Broos CE, Simpson LJ. IFN-γ-producing T-helper 17.1 cells are increased in sarcoidosis and are more prevalent than T-helper type 1 cells. American Journal of Respiratory and Critical Care Medicine. 2016;**193**(11):1281-1291. DOI: 10.1164/rccm.201507-1499OC

[130] Belperio JA, Shaikh F, Abtin F. Extrapulmonary sarcoidosis with a focus on cardiac, nervous system, and ocular involvement. EClinicalMedicine. 2021;**37**:100966. DOI: 10.1016/j.eclinm.2021.100966

[131] Serei VD, Fyfe B. The many faces of cardiac sarcoidosis. American Journal of Clinical Pathology. 2020;**153**(3):294-302. DOI: 10.1093/ajcp/aqz169

[132] Bagwan IN, Hooper LVB, Sheppard MN. Cardiac sarcoidosis and sudden death. The heart may look normal or mimic other cardiomyopathies. Virchows Archiv. 2011;**458**(6):671-678. DOI: 10.1007/s00428-010-1003-8

[133] Patel MR, Cawley PJ, Heitner JF. Detection of myocardial damage in patients with sarcoidosis. Circulation. 2009;**120**(20):1969-1977. DOI: 10.1161/CIRCULATIONAHA.109.851352

[134] Kurmann R, Mankad SV, Mankad R. Echocardiography in sarcoidosis. Current Cardiology Reports. 2018;**20**(11):118. DOI: 10.1007/s11886-018-1065-9

[135] Yafasova A, Fosbøl EL, Schou M. Long-term adverse cardiac outcomes in patients with sarcoidosis. Journal of the American College of Cardiology. 2020;**76**(7):767-777. DOI: 10.1016/j.jacc.2020.06.038

[136] Doughan AR, Williams BR. Cardiac sarcoidosis. Heart (British

Cardiac Society). 2006;**92**(2):282-288. DOI: 10.1136/HRT.2005.080

[137] Terasaki F, Azuma A, Anzai T. JCS 2016 guideline on diagnosis and treatment of cardiac sarcoidosis – Digest version. Circulation Journal. 2019;**83**(11):2329-2388. DOI: 10.1253/circj.CJ-19-0508

[138] Jeudy J, Burke AP, White CS, Kramer GBG, Frazier AA. Cardiac sarcoidosis: The challenge of radiologic-pathologic correlation: From the radiologic pathology archives. Radiographics. 2015;**35**(3):657-679. DOI: 10.1148/rg.2015140247

[139] Oyama-Manabe N, Manabe O, Aikawa T, Tsuneta S. The role of multimodality imaging in cardiac sarcoidosis. Korean Circulation Journal. 2021;**51**(7):561-578. DOI: 10.4070/kcj.2021.0104

[140] Blankstein R, Waller AH. Evaluation of known or suspected cardiac sarcoidosis. Circulation. Cardiovascular Imaging. 2016;**9**(3):e000867. DOI: 10.1161/CIRCIMAGING.113.000867

[141] Okasha O, Kazmirczak F, Chen KA, Farzaneh-Far A, Shenoy C. Myocardial involvement in patients with histologically diagnosed cardiac sarcoidosis: A systematic review and meta-analysis of gross pathological images from autopsy or cardiac transplantation cases. Journal of the American Heart Association. 2019;**8**(10):e011253. DOI: 10.1161/JAHA.118.011253

[142] Youssef G, Beanlands RSB, Birnie DH, Nery PB. Cardiac sarcoidosis: Applications of imaging in diagnosis and directing treatment. Heart. 2011;**97**(24):2078-2087

[143] Ohira H, Tsujino I, Ishimaru S. Myocardial imaging with 18F-fluoro-2-deoxyglucose positron emission tomography and magnetic resonance imaging in sarcoidosis. European Journal of Nuclear Medicine and Molecular Imaging. 2008;**35**(5):933-941

[144] Terasaki F, Kusano K, Nakajima T. The characteristics of Japanese guidelines on diagnosis and treatment of cardiac sarcoidosis compared with the previous guidelines. Sarcoidosis, Vasculitis, and Diffuse Lung Diseases. 2022;**39**(3). DOI: 10.36141/svdld.v39i3.12531

[145] Judson MA, Costabel U, Drent M. The WASOG sarcoidosis organ assessment instrument: An update of a previous clinical tool. Sarcoidosis, Vasculitis, and Diffuse Lung Diseases. 2014;**31**(1):19-27

[146] Lehtonen J, Uusitalo V, Pöyhönen P, Mäyränpää MI, Kupari M. Cardiac sarcoidosis: Phenotypes, diagnosis, treatment, and prognosis. European Heart Journal. 2023;**44**(17):1495-1510. DOI: 10.1093/EURHEARTJ/EHAD067

[147] Grutters JC, van den Bosch JM. Corticosteroid treatment in sarcoidosis. The European Respiratory Journal. 2006;**28**(3):627-636. DOI: 10.1183/09031936.06.00105805

[148] Iannuzzi MC, Rybicki BA, Teirstein AS. Sarcoidosis. The New England Journal of Medicine. 2007;**357**(21):2153-2165. DOI: 10.1056/NEJMra071714

[149] Cheng RK, Kittleson MM, Beavers CJ. Diagnosis and Management of Cardiac Sarcoidosis: A scientific statement from the American Heart Association. Circulation. 2024;**149**(21). DOI: 10.1161/CIR.0000000000001240

[150] Nagai S, Yokomatsu T, Tanizawa K. Treatment with methotrexate and

low-dose corticosteroids in sarcoidosis patients with cardiac lesions. Internal Medicine. 2014;**53**(23). DOI: 10.2169/internalmedicine.53.3120

[151] Rosen NS et al. Cardiac sarcoidosis outcome differences: A comparison of patients with de novo cardiac versus known extracardiac sarcoidosis at presentation. Respiratory Medicine. 2022;**198**:106864. DOI: 10.1016/j.rmed.2022.106864

[152] Fussner LA et al. Management and outcomes of cardiac sarcoidosis: A 20-year experience in two tertiary care centres. European Journal of Heart Failure. 2018;**20**:1713-1720. DOI: 10.1002/ejhf.1319

[153] Velikanova D, Pöyhönen P, Lehtonen J. End-stage heart failure in cardiac sarcoidosis. Circulation. 2024;**149**(11):885-887. DOI: 10.1161/CIRCULATIONAHA.123.066962

[154] Mehra M, Canter CE, Hannan MM. The 2016 International Society for Heart Lung Transplantation listing criteria for heart transplantation: A 10-year update. The Journal of Heart and Lung Transplantation. 2016;**1**:1-23

[155] Crawford TC et al. A contemporary analysis of heart transplantation and bridge-to-transplant mechanical circulatory support outcomes in cardiac sarcoidosis. Journal of Cardiac Failure. 2018;**24**:384-391. DOI: 10.1016/j.cardfail.2018.02.009

[156] Jackson KC et al. Heart transplantation outcomes in cardiac sarcoidosis. The Journal of Heart and Lung Transplantation. 2022;**41**:113-122. DOI: 10.1016/j.healun.2021.08.012

[157] Raeisi-Giglou P, Rodriguez ER, Blackstone EH, Tan CD, Hsich EM. Verification of heart disease: Implications for a new heart transplantation allocation system. JACC. Heart Failure. 2017;**5**:904-913. DOI: 10.1016/j.jchf.2017.09.022

[158] Baughman RP, Drent M, Culver DA. Endpoints for clinical trials of sarcoidosis. Sarcoidosis, Vasculitis, and Diffuse Lung Diseases. 2012;**29**(2):90-98

[159] Hena KM, Patterson KC. Making Progress in clinical trials in sarcoidosis. Chest. 2023;**164**(3):682-685. DOI: 10.1016/j.chest.2023.03.039

[160] Birnie D et al. Cardiac sarcoidosis multi-center randomized controlled trial (CHASM CS-RCT). American Heart Journal. 2020;**220**:246-252. DOI: 10.1016/J.AHJ.2019.10.003

[161] Crownover BK, Covey CJ. Hereditary hemochromatosis. American Family Physician. 2013;**87**(3):183-190

[162] Kremastinos DT, Farmakis D, Aessopos A. β-Thalassemia cardiomyopathy: History, present considerations, and future perspectives. Circulation. Heart Failure. 2010;**3**(3):451-458

[163] Gladwin MT, Sachdev V. Cardiovascular abnormalities in sickle cell disease. Journal of the American College of Cardiology. 2012;**59**(13):1123-1133

[164] Gulati V, Harikrishnan P, Palaniswamy C, Aronow WS, Jain D, Frishman WH. Cardiac involvement in hemochromatosis. Cardiology in Review. 2014;**22**(2):56-68

[165] Aronow WS. Management of cardiac hemochromatosis. Archives of Medical Science. 2018;**14**(3):560-568. DOI: 10.5114/aoms.2017.68729

[166] Ahmed S, Peterson SJ, Parikh MA, Frishman WH. Cardiovascular

manifestations of hemochromatosis: A review of pathophysiology, mechanisms, and treatment options. Cardiology in Review. 2025;**33**(4):359-364. DOI: 10.1097/CRD.0000000000000622

[167] Kang W, Barad A, Clark AG. Ethnic differences in iron status. Advances in Nutrition. 2021;**12**(5):1838-1853. DOI: 10.1093/advances/nmab035

[168] Swinkels DW, Janssen MC, Bergmans J, Marx JJ. Hereditary hemochromatosis: Genetic complexity and new diagnostic approaches. Clinical Chemistry. 2006;**52**(6):950-968. DOI: 10.1373/clinchem.2006.068684

[169] Pietrangelo A. Hereditary hemochromatosis–A new look at an old disease. The New England Journal of Medicine. 2004;**350**:2383-2397

[170] Wood JC. History and current impact of cardiac magnetic resonance imaging on the management of iron overload. Circulation. 2009;**120**:1937-1939

[171] Porter JB. Concepts and goals in the management of transfusional iron overload. American Journal of Hematology. 2007;**82**(12):1136-1139

[172] Jensen PD, Jensen FT, Christensen T, Eiskjaer H, Baandrup U, Nielsen JL. Evaluation of myocardial iron by magnetic resonance imaging during iron chelation therapy with deferrioxamine: Indication of close relation between myocardial iron content and chelatable iron pool. Blood. 2003;**101**:4632-4639

[173] Kremastinos DT, Farmakis D. Iron overload cardiomyopathy in clinical practice. Circulation. 2011;**124**:2253-2263. DOI: 10.1161/CIRCULATIONAHA.111.050773

[174] Carpenter JP et al. On T2* magnetic resonance and cardiac iron. Circulation. 2011;**123**:1519-1528

[175] Murphy CJ, Oudit GY. Iron-overload cardiomyopathy: Pathophysiology, diagnosis, and treatment. Journal of Cardiac Failure. 2010;**16**:888-900

[176] Kremastinos DT, Toutouzas PK, Vyssoulis GP, Venetis CA, Vretou HP, Avgoustakis DG. Global and segmental left ventricular function in beta-thalassemia. Cardiology. 1985;**72**:129-139

[177] Furth PA, Futterweit W, Gorlin R. Refractory biventricular heart failure in secondary hemochromatosis. The American Journal of the Medical Sciences. 1985;**290**:209-213

[178] Gujja P, Rosing DR, Tripodi DJ, Shizukuda Y. Iron overload cardiomyopathy: Better understanding of an increasing disorder. Journal of the American College of Cardiology. 2010;**56**:1001-1012

[179] Wu VC, Huang JW, Wu MS. The effect of iron stores on corrected QT dispersion in patients undergoing peritoneal dialysis. American Journal of Kidney Diseases. 2004;**44**:720-728

[180] Rose RA, Sellan M, Simpson JA. Iron overload decreases CaV1.3-dependent L-type Ca2+ currents leading to bradycardia, altered electrical conduction, and atrial fibrillation. Circulation. Arrhythmia and Electrophysiology. 2011;**118**:174-177

[181] Candore G, Balistreri CR, Lio D. Association between HFE mutations and acute myocardial infarction: A study in patients from northern and southern Italy. Blood Cells, Molecules & Diseases. 2003;**31**:57-62

[182] Kirk P et al. International reproducibility of single breathhold T2*

MR for cardiac and liver iron assessment among five thalassemia centers. Journal of Magnetic Resonance Imaging. 2010;**32**:315-319. DOI: 10.1002/jmri.22245

[183] Alam MH et al. T1 at 1.5T and 3T compared with conventional T2* at 1.5T for cardiac siderosis. Journal of Cardiovascular Magnetic Resonance. 2015;**17**(102). DOI: 10.1186/s12968-015-0207-0

[184] Cooper LT, Baughman KL, Feldman AM. American College of Cardiology, European Society of Cardiology, Heart Failure Society of America, heart failure Association of the European Society of cardiology the role of endomyocardial biopsy in the management of cardiovascular disease a scientific statement from the American Heart Association, the American College of Cardiology, and the European Society of Cardiology Endorsed by the Heart Failure Society of America and the Heart Failure Association of the European Society of Cardiology. Journal of the American College of Cardiology. 2007;**50**(19):1914-1931

[185] Kontoghiorghes GL, Eracleous E, Economides C. Advances in iron overload therapies: Prospects for effective use of deferiprone (L1), deferoxamine, the new experimental chelators ICL670, GT56-252, LINA11 and their combinations. Current Medicinal Chemistry. 2005;**12**:2663-2681

[186] Anderson LJ, Westwood MA, Holden S. Myocardial iron clearance during reversal of siderotic cardiomyopathy with intravenous desferrioxamine: A prospective study using T2* cardiovascular magnetic resonance. British Journal of Haematology. 2004;**127**:348-355

[187] Modell B, Khan M, Darlison M. Survival in beta-thalassemia major in the UK: Data from the UK thalassaemia register. Lancet. 2000;**355**:2051-2052

[188] Pepe A, Rossi G, Capra M. A T2* MRI prospective survey on heart and liver iron in thalassemia major patients treated with deferasirox versus deferiprone and desferrioxamine in monotherapy (abstract 4267). Blood. 2010;**116**:1731

[189] Tanner MA, Galanello R, Dessi C. Combined chelation therapy in thalassemia major for the treatment of severe myocardial siderosis with left ventricular dysfunction. Journal of Cardiovascular Magnetic Resonance. 2008;**10**:12

[190] Kremastinos DT, Tsetsos GA, Tsiapras DP, Karavolias GK, Ladis VA, Kattamis CA. Heart failure in beta thalassemia: A 5-year follow-up study. The American Journal of Medicine. 2001;**111**:349-354

[191] Aessopos A, Berdoukas V, Tsironi M. The heart in transfusion dependent homozygous thalassaemia today–prediction, prevention and management. European Journal of Haematology. 2008;**80**:93-106

[192] Yancy CW, Jessup M, Bozkurt B. "ACCF/AHA guidelines for the management of heart failure: Executive summary. A report of the American College of Cardiology Foundation/American Heart Association task force on practice guidelines. Developed in collaboration with the American College of Chest Physicians, Heart Rhythm Society, and International Society for Heart and Lung Transplantation," endorsed by the American Association of Cardiovascular and Pulmonary Rehabilitation. Journal of the American College of Cardiology. 2013;**62**:1495-1539

[193] Caines AE, Kpodonu J, Massad MG. Cardiac transplantation in patients

with iron overload cardiomyopathy. The Journal of Heart and Lung Transplantation. 2005;**24**:486-488

[194] Kwon YIC et al. Differences in outcomes of combined heart-liver transplantation by primary cardiac diagnosis. JHLT Open. 2024;**6**:100147. DOI: 10.1016/j.jhlto.2024.100147

[195] Robinson MR, Al-Kindi SG, Oliveira GH. Heart and heart-liver transplantation in patients with hemochromatosis. International Journal of Cardiology. 2017;**244**:226-228. DOI: 10.1016/j.ijcard.2017.06.075

[196] Shubin AD, Gregorio L, Hwang C, MacConmara M. Combined heart-liver transplantation in a case of haemochromatosis. BML Case Reports. 2021;**14**(5). DOI: 10.1136/bcr-2020-241508

[197] Jermyn R, Soe E, D'Alessandro D. Cardiac failure after liver transplantation requiring a biventricular assist device. Case Reports in Transplantation. 2014;**2014**:946961

[198] Viatte L, Nicolas G, Lou DQ. Chronic hepcidin induction causes hyposideremia and alters the pattern of cellular iron accumulation in hemochromatotic mice. Blood. 2006;**107**:2952-2958

[199] Kowdley KV, Modi NB, Peltekian K. Rusfertide for the treatment of iron overload in HFE-related haemochromatosis: An open-label, multicentre, proof-of-concept phase 2 trial. The Lancet Gastroenterology & Hepatology. 2023;**8**(12):1118-1128. DOI: 10.1016/S2468-1253(23)00250-9

[200] Thalassemic Iron Overload Cardiomyopathy is Ameliorated by Taurine Supplementation (TICATS). ClinicalTrials.gov. Available from: https://clinicaltrials.gov/study/NCT04291352 [Accessed: September 21, 2025]

[201] Nair V, Belanger EC, Veinot JP. Lysosomal storage disorders affecting the heart: A review. Cardiovascular Pathology. 2019;**39**:12-24. DOI: 10.1016/j.carpath.2018.11.002

[202] Germain DP, Elliott PM, Falissard B. The effect of enzyme replacement therapy on clinical outcomes in male patients with Fabry disease: A systematic literature review by a European panel of experts. Molecular Genetics and Metabolism Reports. 2019;**19**:100454. DOI: 10.1016/j.ymgmr.2019.100454

[203] Pieroni M, Moon JC, Arbustini E. "Cardiac involvement in Fabry disease," JACC review topic of the week. Journal of the American College of Cardiology. 2021;**77**(7):922-936. DOI: 10.1016/j.jacc.2020.12.024

[204] Van Der Veen SJ, Hollak CEM, Van Kuilenburg ABP, Langeveld M. Developments in the treatment of Fabry disease. Journal of Inherited Metabolic Disease. 2020;**43**(5):908-921. DOI: 10.1002/jimd.12228

[205] Zarate YA, Hopkin RJ. Fabry's disease. Lancet. 2008;**372**(9647):1427-1435. DOI: 10.1016/S0140-6736(08)61589-5

[206] Gilchrist M, Casanova F, Tyrrell JS, Cannon S, Wood AR, Fife N. Prevalence of Fabry disease-causing variants in the UK biobank. Journal of Medical Genetics. 2022;**60**(4). DOI: 10.1136/jmg-2022-108523

[207] Spada M, Pagliardini S, Yasuda M, Tukel T, Thiagarajan G, Sakuraba H. High incidence of later-onset Fabry disease revealed by newborn screening*. American Journal

of Human Genetics. 2006;**79**(1):31-40. DOI: 10.1086/504601

[208] Arends M, Wanner C, Hughes D, Mehta A, Oder D, Watkinson OT. Characterization of classical and nonclassical Fabry disease: A multicenter study. Journal of the American Society of Nephrology : JASN. 2017;**28**(5):1631-1641. DOI: 10.1681/ASN.2016090964

[209] Kim WS, Kim HS, Shin J, Park JC, Yoo HW, Takenaka T. Prevalence of Fabry disease in Korean men with left ventricular hypertrophy. Journal of Korean Medical Science. 2019;**34**(7). DOI: 10.3346/jkms.2019.34.e63

[210] Alecek T, Honzikova J, Poupetova H, Vlaskova H, Kuchynka P, Golan L. Prevalence of Fabry disease in male patients with unexplained left ventricular hypertrophy in primary cardiology practice: Prospective Fabry cardiomyopathy screening study (FACSS). Journal of Inherited Metabolic Disease. 2014;**37**(3):455-460. DOI: 10.1007/s10545-013-9659-2

[211] Averbuch T, White JA, Fine NM. Anderson-Fabry disease cardiomyopathy: An update on epidemiology, diagnostic approach, management and monitoring strategies. Frontiers in Cardiovascular Medicine. 2023;**10**:1152568. DOI: 10.3389/fcvm.2023.1152568

[212] Ivanova M. Altered sphingolipids metabolism damaged mitochondrial functions: Lessons learned from Gaucher and Fabry diseases. Journal of Clinical Medicine. 2020;**9**(4). DOI: 10.3390/jcm9041116

[213] Rozenfeld P, Feriozzi S. Contribution of inflammatory pathways to Fabry disease pathogenesis. Molecular Genetics and Metabolism. 2017;**122**(3):19-27. DOI: 10.1016/j.ymgme.2017.09.004

[214] Liu D, Oder D, Salinger T, Hu K, Müntze J, Weidemann F. Association and diagnostic utility of diastolic dysfunction and myocardial fibrosis in patients with Fabry disease. Open Heart. 2018;**5**(2). DOI: 10.1136/openhrt-2018-000803

[215] Akhtar MM, Elliott PM. Anderson-Fabry disease in heart failure. Biophysical Reviews. 2018;**10**(4):1107-1119. DOI: 10.1007/s12551-018-0432-5

[216] Yogasundaram H, Nikhanj A, Chatur S, Qi A, Hagen L, Bailey L. Burden of valvular heart disease in patients with Fabry disease. Journal of the American Society of Echocardiography. 2022;**35**(2):236-238. DOI: 10.1016/j.echo.2021.09.013

[217] Namdar M. Electrocardiographic changes and arrhythmia in Fabry disease. Frontiers in Cardiovascular Medicine. 2016;**3**(7). DOI: 10.3389/fcvm.2016.00007

[218] Perry R, Shah R, Saiedi M. The Role of Cardiac Imaging in the Diagnosis and Management of Anderson-Fabry Disease [Published Correction Appears in JACC Cardiovasc Imaging]. 2019. DOI: 10.1016/j.jcmg.2019.07.004

[219] Nordin S, Kozor R, Medina-Menacho K. Proposed stages of myocardial phenotype development in Fabry disease. JACC: Cardiovascular Imaging. 2019;**12**(8):1673-1683. DOI: 10.1016/j.jcmg.2018.03.020

[220] Ortiz A et al. Fabry disease revisited: Management and treatment recommendations for adult patients. Molecular Genetics and Metabolism. 2018;**123**(4):416-427. DOI: 10.1016/j.ymgme.2018.02.014

[221] Lee CL, Lin SP, Niu DM, Lin HY. Fabry disease and the effectiveness of enzyme replacement therapy (ERT)

in left ventricular hypertrophy (LVH) improvement: A review and meta-analysis. International Journal of Medical Sciences. 2022;**19**(1):126-131. DOI: 10.7150/ijms.66448

[222] Weidemann F, Niemann M, Breunig F, Herrmann S, Beer M, Störk S. Long-term effects of enzyme replacement therapy on Fabry cardiomyopathy: Evidence for a better outcome with early treatment. Circulation. 2009;**119**(4):524-529. DOI: 10.1161/CIRCULATIONAHA.108.794529

[223] Lenders M, Brand E. Effects of enzyme replacement therapy and antidrug antibodies in patients with Fabry disease. JASN. 2018;**29**(9):2265-2278. DOI: 10.1681/ASN.2018030329

[224] Ruderfer I, Shulman A, Kizhner T, Azulay Y, Nataf Y, Tekoah Y. Development and analytical characterization of pegunigalsidase alfa, a chemically cross-linked plant recombinant human α-galactosidase-a for treatment of Fabry disease. Bioconjugate Chemistry. 2018;**29**(5):1630-1639. DOI: 10.1021/acs.bioconjchem.8b00133

[225] Rombach SM, Aerts JMFG, Poorthuis BJHM, Groener JEM, Donker-Koopman W, Hendriks E. Long-term effect of antibodies against infused alpha-galactosidase a in Fabry disease on plasma and urinary (lyso)Gb3 reduction and treatment outcome. PLoS One. 2012;**7**(10). DOI: 10.1371/journal.pone.0047805

[226] Mauhin W, Lidove O, Amelin D, Lamari F, Caillaud C, Mingozzi F. Deep characterization of the anti-drug antibodies developed in Fabry disease patients, a prospective analysis from the French multicenter cohort FFABRY. Orphanet Journal of Rare Diseases. 2018;**13**(1). DOI: 10.1186/s13023-018-0877-4

[227] Benjamin ER, Della Valle MC, Wu X, Katz E, Pruthi F, Bond S. The validation of pharmacogenetics for the identification of Fabry patients to be treated with migalastat. Genetics in Medicine. 2017;**19**(4):430-438. DOI: 10.1038/gim.2016.122

[228] Hughes DA, Nicholls K, Shankar SP, Sunder-Plassmann G, Koeller D, Nedd K. Oral pharmacological chaperone migalastat compared with enzyme replacement therapy in Fabry disease: 18-month results from the randomised phase III ATTRACT study. Journal of Medical Genetics. 2017;**54**(4):288-296. DOI: 10.1136/jmedgenet-2016-104178

[229] Camporeale A, Bandera F, Pieroni M, et al. Effect of Migalastat on cArdiac InvOlvement in FabRry DiseAse: MAIORA study. Journal of Medical Genetics. 2023;**60**(9):850-858. DOI: 10.1136/jmg-2022-108768

[230] Mehra MR et al. International Society for Heart Lung Transplantation (ISHLT) infectious diseases, Pediatric and heart failure and transplantation councils. The 2016 International Society for Heart Lung Transplantation listing criteria for heart transplantation: A 10-year update. The Journal of Heart and Lung Transplantation. 2016;**35**:1-23. DOI: 10.1016/j.healun.2015.10.023

[231] Kyem G, Okorozo A, Hamdan H, Tuffaha AM. A case report of kidney after heart transplant in patient with Fabry disease. Transplantation Proceedings. 2023;**55**(8):1975-1977. DOI: 10.1016/j.transproceed.2023.07.009

[232] Verocai F, Clarke JT, Iwanochko RM. Case report: Long-term outcome post-heart transplantation in a woman with Fabry's disease. Journal of Inherited

Metabolic Disease. 2010;**33**(Suppl. 3):S385-S387. DOI: 10.1007/s10545-010-9194-3

[233] Di Nora C, Livi U. Heart transplantation in cardiac storage diseases: Data on Fabry disease and cardiac amyloidosis. Current Opinion in Organ Transplantation. 2020;**25**(3):211-217. DOI: 10.1097/MOT.0000000000000756

[234] Wanner C, Kimonis V, Politei J. Understanding and modifying Fabry disease: Rationale and design of a pivotal phase 3 study and results from a patient-reported outcome validation study. Molecular Genetics and Metabolism Reports. 2022;**31**:100862. DOI: 10.1016/j.ymgmr.2022.100862

[235] Domm JM, Wootton SK, Medin JA, West ML. Gene therapy for Fabry disease: Progress, challenges, and outlooks on gene-editing. Molecular Genetics and Metabolism. 2021;**134**(1):117-131. DOI: 10.1016/j.ymgme.2021.07.006

[236] Zhu X, Yin L, Theisen M, Zhuo J, Siddiqui S, Levy B. Systemic mRNA therapy for the treatment of Fabry disease: Preclinical studies in wild-type mice, Fabry mouse model, and wild-type non-human primates. American Journal of Human Genetics. 2019;**104**(4):625-637. DOI: 10.1016/j.ajhg.2019.02.003

[237] Ter Huurne M et al. GLA-modified RNA treatment lowers GB3 levels in iPSC-derived cardiomyocytes from Fabry-affected individuals. The American Journal of Human Genetics. 2023;**110**(9):1600-1605. DOI: 10.1016/j.ajhg.2023.07.013

[238] Yang Z et al. Danon disease as an Underrecognized cause of hypertrophic cardiomyopathy in children. Circulation. 2005;**112**(11):1612-1617. DOI: 10.1161/CIRCULATIONAHA.105.546481

[239] Takahashi M et al. Germline mosaicism of a novel mutation in lysosome-associated membrane protein-2 deficiency (Danon disease). Annals of Neurology. 2002;**52**(1):122-125. DOI: 10.1002/ana.10235

[240] Wang Y, Jia M, Guo Y, Zhang T, Ning B. Case report: Danon disease: Six family members and literature review. Frontiers in Cardiovascular Medicine. 2022;**9**:842282. DOI: 10.3389/fcvm.2022.842282

[241] Hong KN, Eshraghian EA, Arad M. "International consensus on differential diagnosis and Management of Patients with Danon Disease," JACC state-of-the-art review. Journal of the American College of Cardiology. 2023;**82**(16):1628-1647. DOI: 10.1016/j.jacc.2023.08.014

[242] Charron P et al. Danon's disease as a cause of hypertrophic cardiomyopathy: A systematic survey. Heart. 2004;**90**(8):842-846

[243] Brambatti M, Caspi O, Maolo A. Danon disease: Gender differences in presentation and outcomes. International Journal of Cardiology. 2019;**286**:92-98. DOI: 10.1016/j.ijcard.2019.01.020

[244] Endo Y, Furuta A, Nishino I. Danon disease: A phenotypic expression of LAMP-2 deficiency. Acta Neuropathologica. 2015;**129**(3):391-398. DOI: 10.1007/s00401-015-1385-4

[245] Alcalai R et al. LAMP2 cardiomyopathy: Consequences of impaired autophagy in the heart. Journal of the American Heart Association. 2021;**10**(17):e018829. DOI: 10.1161/JAHA.120.018829

[246] Samad F et al. Malignant cardiac phenotypic expression of Danon disease

(LAMP2 cardiomyopathy). International Journal of Cardiology. 2017;**245**:201-206. DOI: 10.1016/j.ijcard.2017.06.031

[247] Jhaveri S, Herber J, Zahka K, Boyle GJ, Saarel EV, Aziz PF. Arrhythmias and fasciculoventricular pathways in patients with Danon disease: A single center experience. Journal of Cardiovascular Electrophysiology. 2019;**30**(10):1932-1938. DOI: 10.1111/jce.14049

[248] Stevens-Lapsley JE, Kramer LR, Balter JE, Jirikowic J, Boucek D, Taylor M. Functional performance and muscle strength phenotypes in men and women with Danon disease. Muscle and Nerve. 2010;**42**(6):908-914. DOI: 10.1002/mus.21811

[249] Prall FR et al. Ophthalmic manifestations of Danon disease. Ophthalmology. 2006;**113**(6):1010-1013. DOI: 10.1016/j.ophtha.2006.02.030

[250] Wei X et al. Cardiac phenotype characterization at MRI in patients with Danon disease: A retrospective multicenter case series. Radiology. 2021;**299**:303-310. DOI: 10.1148/radiol.2021203996

[251] Miani D et al. Sudden death associated with danon disease in women. The American Journal of Cardiology. 2012;**109**(3):406-411

[252] Balmer C et al. Familial X-linked cardiomyopathy (Danon disease): Diagnostic confirmation by mutation analysis of the LAMP2 gene. European Journal of Pediatrics. 2005;**164**(8):509-514

[253] Nishino I et al. Primary LAMP-2 deficiency causes X-linked vacuolar cardiomyopathy and myopathy (Danon disease). Nature. 2000;**406**(6798):906-910

[254] D'souza RS et al. Danon disease: Clinical features, evaluation, and management. Circulation. Heart Failure. 2014;7(5):843-849

[255] Hong KN, Battikha C, John S. Cardiac transplantation in Danon disease. Journal of Cardiac Failure. 2022;**28**(4):664-669. DOI: 10.1016/j.cardfail.2021.11.007

[256] Prondzynski M, Mearini G, Carrier L. Gene therapy strategies in the treatment of hypertrophic cardiomyopathy. Pflügers Archiv - European Journal of Physiology. 2019;**471**(5):807-815. DOI: 10.1007/s00424-018-2173-5

[257] Gene Therapy for Male Patients With Danon Disease (DD) Using RP-A501; AAV9.LAMP2B. ClinicalTrials.gov. Available from: https://clinicaltrials.gov/study/NCT03882437 [Accessed: September 21, 2025]

[258] Tuohy CV, Kaul S, Song HK, Nazer B, Heitner SB. Hypertrophic cardiomyopathy: The future of treatment. European Journal of Heart Failure. 2020;**22**(2):228-240. DOI: 10.1002/ejhf.1715

[259] Teener J. Late-onset Pompe's disease. Seminars in Neurology. 2013;**32**(5):506-511. DOI: 10.1055/s-0033-1334469

[260] Kishnani PS, Steiner RD. Pompe disease diagnosis and management guideline. Genetics in Medicine. 2006;**8**(5):267-288. DOI: 10.1097/01.gim.0000218152.87434.f3

[261] Lee DH, Qiu WJ, Lee J, Chien YH, Hwu WL. Hypertrophic cardiomyopathy in pompe disease is not limited to the classic infantile-onset phenotype. JIMD Reports. 2014;**17**:71-75. DOI: 10.1007/8904_2014_339

[262] Stevens D, Milani-Nejad S, Mozaffar T. Pompe disease: A clinical, diagnostic, and therapeutic overview. Current Treatment Options in Neurology. 2022;**24**(11):573-588. DOI: 10.1007/s11940-022-00736-1

[263] Fayssoil A. Cardiomyopathy in Pompe's disease. European Journal of Internal Medicine. 2008;**19**(1):57-59. DOI: 10.1016/j.ejim.2007.09.018

[264] Lim JA, Li L, Raben N. Pompe disease: From pathophysiology to therapy and back again. Frontiers in Aging Neuroscience. 2014;**6**(177)

[265] Nagueh SF, Bachinski LL, Meyer D. Tissue Doppler imaging consistently detects myocardial abnormalities in patients with hypertrophic cardiomyopathy and provides a novel means for an early diagnosis before and independently of hypertrophy. Circulation. 2001;**104**(2):128-130. DOI: 10.1161/01.cir.104.2.128

[266] Limongelli G, Fratta F. S1.4 Cardiovascular involvement in Pompe disease. Acta Myologica. 2011;**30**(3):202-203

[267] Forsha D, Li JS, Smith PB. Cardiovascular abnormalities in late-onset Pompe disease and response to enzyme replacement therapy. Genetics in Medicine. 2011;**13**(7):625-631. DOI: 10.1097/GIM.0b013e3182142966

[268] Wokke JH, Escolar DM, Pestronk A. Clinical features of late-onset Pompe disease: A prospective cohort study. Muscle & Nerve. 2008;**38**(4):1236-1245. DOI: 10.1002/mus.21025

[269] Colburn R, Lapidus D. An analysis of Pompe newborn screening data: A new prevalence at birth, insight and discussion. Frontiers in Pediatrics. 2024;**11**:1221140. DOI: 10.3389/fped.2023.1221140

[270] Kishnani PS, Corzo D, Nicolino M, Byrne B, Mandel H, Hwu WL. Recombinant human acid [alpha]-glucosidase: Major clinical benefits in infantile-onset Pompe disease. Neurology. 2007;**68**(2):99-109

[271] Harlaar L, Hogrel JY, Perniconi B, Kruijshaar ME, Rizopoulos D, Taouagh N. Large variation in effects during 10 years of enzyme therapy in adults with Pompe disease. Neurology. 2019;**93**(19)

[272] Diaz-Manera J, Kishnani PS, Kushlaf H, Ladha S, Mozaffar T, Straub V. Safety and efficacy of avalglucosidase alfa versus alglucosidase alfa in patients with late-onset Pompe disease (COMET): A phase 3, randomised, multicentre trial. Lancet Neurology. 2021;**20**(12):1012-1026

[273] Schoser B, Roberts M, Byrne BJ, Sitaraman S, Jiang H, Laforêt P. Safety and efficacy of cipaglucosidase alfa plus miglustat versus alglucosidase alfa plus placebo in late-onset Pompe disease (PROPEL): An international, randomised, double-blind, parallel-group, phase 3 trial. Lancet Neurology. 2021;**20**(12):1027-1037

[274] FDA Approves Nexviazyme® (avalglucosidase alfa-ngpt), An Important New Treatment Option for Late-Onset Pompe Disease - Sanofi. Available from: www.sanofi.com, https://www.sanofi.com/en/media-room/press-releases/2021/2021-08-06-15-42-21-2276588

[275] Blair HA. Cipaglucosidase alfa: First approval. Drugs. 2023;**83**(8):739-745. DOI: 10.1007/s40265-023-01886-5

[276] Asklepios Biopharmaceutical, Inc. A Phase 1 Study of the Safety of AAV2/8-LSPhGAA (ACTUS-101) in Late-Onset Pompe Disease.

clinicaltrials.gov. Clinical trial registration NCT03533673. 2023. [Online]. Available from: https://clinicaltrials.gov/study/NCT03533673 [Accessed: December 18, 2024]

[277] Spark Therapeutics, Inc. Phase 1/2, Dose-Escalation Study to Evaluate the Safety, Tolerability and Efficacy of a Single Intravenous Infusion of SPK-3006 in Adults with Late-Onset Pompe Disease. 2024. clinicaltrials.gov, Clinical trial registration NCT04093349. [Online]. Available from: https://clinicaltrials.gov/study/NCT04093349 [Accessed: December 18, 2024]

[278] Ding E, Hu H, Hodges BL, Migone F, Serra D, Xu F. Efficacy of gene therapy for a prototypical lysosomal storage disease (GSD-II) is critically dependent on vector dose, transgene promoter, and the tissues targeted for vector transduction. Molecular Therapy. 2002;**5**(4):436-446

[279] Kishnani PS, Koeberl DD. Liver depot gene therapy for Pompe disease. Annals of Translational Medicine. 2019;**7**(13)

[280] Astellas Gene Therapies. A Phase 1/2, Open-Label, Ascending-Dose Clinical Study to Evaluate the Safety and Preliminary Efficacy of AT845, an AAV8-Delivered Gene Transfer Therapy in Patients with Late Onset Pompe Disease. clinicaltrials.gov, Clinical trial registration NCT04174105. 2024. [Online]. Available from: https://clinicaltrials.gov/study/NCT04174105 [Accessed: December 18, 2024]

[281] Ullman J. Results from a First in Human Study of MZE001, an Orally Bioavailable Inhibitor of Glycogen Synthase 1 and Potential Substrate Reduction Therapy for Pompe Disease. [Online]. Available from: https://mazetx.com/wp-content/uploads/2023/02/Ullman_20220226_MZE001-Phase-1_Pompe_SRT_GYS1_FINAL.pdf

[282] Hanson E, Sheldon M, Pacheco B, Alkubeysi M, Raizada V. Heart disease in Friedreich's ataxia. World Journal of Cardiology. 2019;**11**(1):1-12. DOI: 10.4330/wjc.v11.i1.1

[283] Michael S et al. Iron and iron-responsive proteins in the cardiomyopathy of Friedreich's ataxia. Cerebellum. 2006;**5**(4):257-267. DOI: 10.1080/14734220600913246

[284] Koeppen AH. Friedreich's ataxia: Pathology, pathogenesis, and molecular genetics. Journal of the Neurological Sciences. 2011;**303**(1):1-12. DOI: 10.1016/j.jns.2011.01.010

[285] Campuzano V et al. Frataxin is reduced in Friedreich ataxia patients and is associated with mitochondrial membranes. Human Molecular Genetics. 1997;**6**:1771-1780

[286] Tsou AY et al. Mortality in Friedreich ataxia. Journal of the Neurological Sciences. 2011;**307**:46-49

[287] Pousset F et al. A 22-year follow-up study of long-term cardiac outcome and predictors of survival in Friedreich ataxia. JAMA Neurology. 2015;**72**:1334-1341

[288] Bidichandani SI, Delatycki MB. Friedreich Ataxia. Seattle WA: University of Washington; 1998

[289] Yilmaz MB, Koç AF, Kasap H, Güzel AI, Sarica Y, Süleymanova D. GAA repeat polymorphism in Turkish Friedreich's ataxia patients. The International Journal of Neuroscience. 2006;**116**(5):565-574

[290] Zhu D, Burke C, Leslie A, Nicholson GA. Friedreich's ataxia

with chorea and myoclonus caused by a compound heterozygosity for a novel deletion and the trinucleotide GAA expansion. Movement Disorders. 2002;**17**(3):585-589

[291] Aranca TV et al. Emerging therapies in Friedreich's ataxia. Neurodegenerative Disease Management. 2016;**6**(1):49-65

[292] Williams CT, Jesus O. Friedreich Ataxia. In: StatPearls. Treasure Island FL: StatPearls Publishing; 2023

[293] Koeppen AH, Ramirez RL, Becker AB. The pathogenesis of cardiomyopathy in Friedreich ataxia. PLoS One. 2015;**10**(3). DOI: 10.1371/journal.pone.0116396

[294] Drysdale J, Arosio P, Invernizzi R, Cazzola M, Volz A. Mitochondrial ferritin: A new player in iron metabolism. Blood Cells, Molecules & Diseases. 2002;**29**:376-383

[295] Marian AJ, Braunwald E. Hypertrophic cardiomyopathy: Genetics, pathogenesis, clinical manifestations, diagnosis, and therapy. Circulation Research. 2017;**121**(7):749-770. DOI: 10.1161/CIRCRESAHA.117.311059

[296] Delatycki MB, Corben LA. Clinical features of Friedreich ataxia. Journal of Child Neurology. 2012;**27**(9):1133-1137

[297] McMurray JJV et al. Effects of candesartan in patients with chronic heart failure and reduced left-ventricular systolic function taking angiotensin-converting-enzyme inhibitors: The CHARM-added trial. Lancet. 2003;**362**(9386):767-771. DOI: 10.1016/S0140-6736(03)14283-3

[298] Solomon SD et al. Influence of ejection fraction on cardiovascular outcomes in a broad spectrum of heart failure patients. Circulation. 2005;**112**(24):3738-3744. DOI: 10.1161/CIRCULATIONAHA.105.561423

[299] Takazaki KAG et al. Pre-clinical left ventricular myocardial remodeling in patients with Friedreich's ataxia: A cardiac MRI study. PLoS One. 2021;**16**(3):e0246633. DOI: 10.1371/journal.pone.0246633

[300] American College of Cardiology Foundation Task Force on Expert Consensus Documents et al. ACCF/ACR/AHA/NASCI/SCMR 2010 expert consensus document on cardiovascular magnetic resonance: A report of the American College of Cardiology Foundation task force on expert consensus documents. Journal of the American College of Cardiology. 2010;**55**(23):2614-2662. DOI: 10.1016/j.jacc.2009.11.011

[301] Peverill RE, Romanelli G, Donelan L, Hassam R, Corben LA, Delatycki MB. Left ventricular structural and functional changes in Friedreich ataxia - relationship with body size, sex, age and genetic severity. PLoS One. 2019;**14**(11):e0225147. DOI: 10.1371/journal.pone.0225147

[302] McCormick A, Shinnick J, Schadt K. Cardiac transplantation in Friedreich ataxia: Extended follow-up. Journal of the Neurological Sciences. 2017;**375**:471-473. DOI: 10.1016/j.jns.2017.01.027

[303] Valero MJ, Muñoz-Blanco JL, Sanchez AG. Should advanced Friedreich's Ataxia be a contraindication for heart transplantation? A case report of a successful procedure in a 58-year-old patient. Journal of Cardiovascular Development and Disease. 2022;**9**(3). DOI: 10.3390/jcdd9030080

[304] Ivak P, Zumrová A, Netuka I. Friedreich's ataxia and advanced heart failure: An ethical conundrum

in decision-making. The Journal of Heart and Lung Transplantation. 2016;**35**(9):1144-1145. DOI: 10.1016/j.healun.2016.06.021

[305] Perdomini M, Belbellaa B, Monassier L, Reutenauer L, Messaddeq N. Prevention and reversal of severe mitochondrial cardiomyopathy by gene therapy in a mouse model of Friedreich's ataxia. Nature Medicine. 2014;**20**:542-547. DOI: 10.1038/nm.3510

[306] Jones SA, Scheller J, Rose-John S. Therapeutic strategies for the clinical blockade of IL-6/gp130 signaling. The Journal of Clinical Investigation. 2011;**121**(9):3375-3383. DOI: 10.1172/JCI57158

[307] Weill Medical College of Cornell University. Phase IA and IB Study of AAVrh.10hFXN Gene Therapy for the Cardiomyopathy of Friedreich's Ataxia. clinicaltrials.gov, Clinical trial registration NCT05302271, 2024. [Online]. Available from: https://clinicaltrials.gov/study/NCT05302271 [Accessed: December 18, 2024]

[308] Retrotope, Inc. A Randomized, Double-Blind, Controlled Study to Assess the Safety, Tolerability, and Pharmacokinetics of RT001 in Patients with Friedreich's Ataxia. clinicaltrials.gov, Clinical trial registration NCT02445794. 2020. [Online]. Available from: https://clinicaltrials.gov/study/NCT02445794 [Accessed: December 18, 2024]

Chapter 3

Takotsubo Cardiomyopathy: A Comprehensive Overview

Andrew Ndakotsu

Abstract

Takotsubo cardiomyopathy (TTC), also known as stress-induced cardiomyopathy or broken heart syndrome, is a transient left ventricular dysfunction often triggered by emotional or physical stress. Although it mimics acute coronary syndrome (ACS) with symptoms such as chest pain, ECG changes, and elevated cardiac biomarkers, TTC is distinguished by the absence of obstructive coronary artery disease. The exact pathophysiology remains unclear, but proposed mechanisms include catecholamine surge, microvascular dysfunction, and coronary artery spasm. Imaging modalities such as echocardiography and cardiac magnetic resonance imaging (MRI) play a pivotal role in diagnosis, with apical ballooning and absence of late gadolinium enhancement (LGE) serving as hallmark features. Management is primarily supportive, with a focus on treating heart failure, preventing thromboembolic complications, and addressing psychological stressors. While most patients recover within weeks, recurrence and long-term complications such as arrhythmias and heart failure remain concerns. Future research aims to refine risk stratification, biomarker discovery, and targeted therapies to improve outcomes. Given the increasing recognition of TTC in clinical practice, an integrated approach involving cardiology, neurology, and psychiatry is essential for comprehensive care.

Keywords: Takotsubo cardiomyopathy, stress-induced cardiomyopathy, acute coronary syndrome, catecholamine surge, cardiac imaging, left ventricular dysfunction

1. Introduction

Takotsubo cardiomyopathy (TTC), also known as stress-induced cardiomyopathy or broken heart syndrome, is a fascinating and complex cardiac condition. It is characterized by a sudden and temporary weakening of the left ventricle (LV), the heart's main pumping chamber, often triggered by severe emotional or physical stress [1]. This condition presents similarly to acute coronary syndrome (ACS), with symptoms such as chest pain and shortness of breath, but it notably lacks the obstructive coronary artery disease (CAD) typically seen in ACS [2]. First described in Japan in 1990 by Sato et al., the syndrome derives its name from the Japanese word "takotsubo," which refers to a ceramic pot used to trap octopuses [3]. This name was chosen because the left ventricle of the heart takes on a shape resembling this pot during the acute phase of the syndrome, a phenomenon known as left ventricle apical ballooning [4]. The condition gained wider recognition in the early 2000s, particularly after a significant earthquake in Niigata Prefecture, Japan, in 2004. Following the earthquake, a notable number of cases were reported, drawing international attention to the syndrome. Consequently earthquakes in New Zealand also have been associated with increased rates of Takotsubo cardiomyopathy [5]. In 2015, the *New England Journal of Medicine* published a paper on TTC, which helped to further establish its recognition and understanding in the medical community [1].

The pathophysiology of TTC is not entirely understood, but it is believed that a surge of stress hormones, such as adrenaline, plays a crucial role [6]. These hormones can "stun" the heart, leading to changes in the heart muscle cells or coronary blood vessels that impair the left ventricle's ability to contract effectively [2]. This condition is more prevalent in postmenopausal women, with over 90% of reported cases occurring in women aged 58–75 [7, 8]. Despite its dramatic presentation, TTC is usually a transient condition, and most patients recover fully with appropriate medical care. However, it can lead to serious complications such as heart failure, arrhythmias, and, in rare cases, death [7, 8]. The diagnosis of TTC is typically confirmed through imaging studies, such as echocardiography or cardiac MRI, which reveal the characteristic LV apical ballooning [9].

Today, TTC is recognized worldwide, and ongoing research continues to explore its pathophysiology, triggers, and treatment options. The syndrome serves as a poignant reminder of the powerful connection between emotional stress and physical health. The condition is relatively rare, but its incidence appears to be increasing, likely due to greater awareness and improved diagnostic techniques.

Several risk factors have been associated with the development of TTC:

1. Gender and age: As mentioned, postmenopausal women are at the highest risk. Hormonal changes after menopause may play a role in this increased susceptibility.

2. Emotional or physical stress: TTC is often triggered by intense emotional or physical stress. Common triggers include the death of a loved one, severe illness, or major surgery.

3. Neurological disorders: Conditions such as subarachnoid hemorrhage and seizures have been linked to an increased risk of TTC.

4. Psychiatric disorders: Anxiety, depression, and other psychiatric conditions are also considered risk factors.

5. Chronic medical conditions: Patients with chronic conditions like hypertension and diabetes may have a higher risk of developing TTC [10].

2. Pathophysiology of Takotsubo cardiomyopathy (TTC)

The exact pathophysiology of TTC is not fully understood, but several mechanisms have been proposed:

- Catecholamine surge: A significant increase in stress hormones, particularly catecholamines like adrenaline, is believed to play a central role. These hormones can cause direct myocardial toxicity, leading to transient LV dysfunction [11].

- Microvascular dysfunction: Stress-induced microvascular dysfunction may impair coronary blood flow, contributing to myocardial stunning and the characteristic apical ballooning [11].

- Coronary artery spasm: Transient spasm of the coronary arteries can reduce blood supply to the myocardium, mimicking the effects of a heart attack without actual blockage [11].

- Myocardial metabolism: Alterations in myocardial metabolism and energy utilization during stress may also contribute to the development of TTC [11, 12].

3. Clinical presentation of TTC

The clinical presentation of TTC often mimics that of acute coronary syndrome (ACS), making it challenging to distinguish between the two without further diagnostic testing. Key clinical features include:

- Chest pain: The most common presenting symptom is acute chest pain, similar to that experienced during a heart attack [1].

- Dyspnea: Shortness of breath is another frequent symptom, reflecting the heart's reduced pumping ability.

- Electrocardiogram (ECG) changes: Patients often exhibit ECG changes, such as ST-segment elevation or T-wave inversion, which are also seen in myocardial infarction [12].

- Elevated cardiac biomarkers: Blood tests may show elevated levels of cardiac biomarkers like troponin, indicating myocardial injury [1, 6, 7].

- Echocardiography findings: Imaging studies, particularly echocardiography, reveal the hallmark feature of TTC apical ballooning of the LV with basal hyperkinesis [9, 11, 12]

- Absence of obstructive CAD: Coronary angiography typically shows no significant obstructive coronary artery disease, distinguishing TTC from ACS [2, 4, 5, 8, 9]

Patients with TTC may also present with less common symptoms such as palpitations, nausea, vomiting, syncope, or, in severe cases, cardiogenic shock. The condition is often preceded by a significant emotional or physical stressor, occurring in approximately two-thirds of cases [1, 6, 10, 13].

4. Diagnostic criteria and workup

TTC, also known as stress-induced cardiomyopathy or broken heart syndrome, requires a comprehensive diagnostic approach to distinguish it from other cardiac conditions, particularly ACS. The diagnostic criteria and workup for TTC involve a combination of clinical evaluation, imaging studies, and laboratory tests.

4.1 Diagnostic criteria

The most widely accepted diagnostic criteria for TTC are the *Revised Mayo Clinic Criteria*, which include the following:

1. Transient left ventricular dysfunction: This includes apical ballooning or mid-ventricular, basal, or focal wall motion abnormalities that extend beyond a single coronary artery distribution.

2. Absence of obstructive coronary artery disease: Coronary angiography should show no significant obstructive coronary artery disease or acute plaque rupture.

3. New electrocardiographic abnormalities: These may include ST-segment elevation, T-wave inversion, or modest elevation of cardiac biomarkers such as troponin.

4. Absence of pheochromocytoma and myocarditis: These conditions must be excluded through appropriate testing [14].

4.2 Workup

The workup for TTC involves several steps to confirm the diagnosis and rule out other conditions:

1. Clinical assessment: A thorough history and physical examination are essential. The clinician should inquire about recent emotional or physical stressors, which are common triggers for TTC [1, 14]

2. Electrocardiogram (ECG): The electrocardiogram (ECG) findings in Takotsubo syndrome can vary widely:

    - Initial presentation: The ECG may appear normal, show nonspecific ST- and T-wave changes, or demonstrate Q waves and ST-segment elevation. ST-segment elevation is more commonly observed in precordial leads and is less frequently accompanied by inferior reciprocal ST-segment depression compared to anterior ST-elevation myocardial infarction (MI) [1].

    - Progression: Within 24–48 hours, the ECG often develops a markedly prolonged QT interval and deep T-wave inversions in both precordial and limb leads. The QT interval prolongation typically improves within a few days, but T-wave abnormalities can persist for weeks to months [4, 8, 9].

5. Cardiac enzymes

Troponin elevation in TTS is typically mild to moderate despite the presence of significant left ventricular (LV) dysfunction. Unlike AMI, where troponin release is driven by myocyte necrosis due to prolonged ischemia, the myocardial injury in TTS is largely due to stress-induced catecholamine toxicity, microvascular dysfunction, and myocardial stunning [6]. This results in a disproportionately low troponin elevation relative to the extent of LV systolic impairment. Studies have reported that mean troponin I levels in TTS often range between 0.1 and 1.0 ng/mL, significantly lower than the markedly elevated levels seen in STEMI, where troponin I can exceed 5–100 ng/mL, depending on infarct size [1]. The relatively lower troponin release in TTS reflects the absence of transmural infarction, as the myocardial dysfunction is typically reversible with supportive care [4].

Some studies suggest that patients with higher troponin levels in TTS may have a greater degree of microvascular injury or direct myocyte damage from extreme catecholamine surges [1]. However, persistently rising or excessively elevated troponin levels should prompt clinicians to reconsider the diagnosis, as conditions like acute coronary syndrome (ACS), myocarditis, or myocardial infarction with non-obstructive coronary arteries (MINOCA) may present with overlapping features [6]. Therefore, troponin trends, along with clinical presentation, ECG changes, and imaging findings (such as apical ballooning on echocardiography or cardiac MRI evidence of myocardial edema without late gadolinium enhancement), are crucial in differentiating TTS from other acute cardiac conditions [11].

TTC is associated with several biomarkers beyond troponin, reflecting myocardial stress, inflammation, and cardiac dysfunction [11]. Natriuretic peptides, including BNP and NT-proBNP, are frequently elevated in TTC, often surpassing levels seen in ACS [1]. The BNP/troponin ratio is notably higher in TTC, aiding differentiation from ACS. Inflammatory markers such as C-reactive protein (CRP) and interleukins (IL-6, IL-8) are often increased, suggesting a systemic inflammatory response [11].

Cardiac stress and injury markers also play a role. Growth Differentiation Factor-15 (GDF-15) and Heart-Type Fatty Acid Binding Protein (H-FABP) have been identified as potential diagnostic tools, while endothelial stress markers like soluble suppression of tumorigenicity-2 (sST2) and soluble urokinase plasminogen activator receptor (suPAR) are elevated in some TTC cases. Heat Shock Protein 70 (HSP70) has emerged as a novel biomarker, with increased levels in TTC compared to non-ST-elevation myocardial infarction NSTEMI [6].

Furthermore, emerging research highlights the role of microRNAs (miR-16 and miR-26a) in TTC, offering insights into its pathophysiology and potential as future diagnostic markers. These biomarkers provide valuable information for distinguishing TTC from other cardiac conditions, but further studies are needed to standardize their clinical use [6].

6. Imaging modalities

6.1 Imaging and left ventricular dysfunction in Takotsubo syndrome

TTS primarily affects the apical and midventricular segments while sparing the basal segments. This unique pattern results in a characteristic apical ballooning appearance, which resembles a Japanese takotsubo (octopus trap), giving the syndrome its name [1, 14]. Unlike AMI, where myocardial necrosis leads to permanent damage, TTS is a reversible cardiomyopathy with functional recovery typically occurring within days to weeks [4, 10]. Imaging plays a central role in diagnosing TTS, differentiating it from AMI and other cardiomyopathies, and assessing the severity of LV dysfunction and potential complications [9, 14].

6.2 Echocardiography: A first-line diagnostic tool

Echocardiography is the first-line imaging modality in suspected TTS due to its widespread availability, rapid assessment capabilities, and ability to detect the hallmark regional wall motion abnormalities (RWMAs) [1, 9]. The classic echocardiographic finding in TTS is apical and midventricular akinesis or hypokinesis with basal hyperkinesis [1, 9, 14]. This pattern is distinct from AMI, where RWMAs typically follow a coronary artery distribution. In TTS, the wall motion abnormalities extend beyond a single coronary vascular territory, reinforcing the diagnosis [1, 9, 11, 14].

In addition to LV dysfunction, echocardiography can reveal several secondary findings that are clinically important. One such finding is dynamic left ventricular outflow tract (LVOT) obstruction, which occurs in approximately 20% of TTS cases due to hypercontractility of the basal myocardium [1, 9, 11, 14]. This obstruction can contribute to hemodynamic instability and cardiogenic shock, making it an essential aspect of echocardiographic evaluation [1, 4, 9, 14]. Another critical finding is mitral regurgitation (MR), which can occur due to tethering of the mitral valve apparatus or systolic anterior motion (SAM) of the mitral valve in cases with LVOT obstruction [1, 4, 9, 11, 14]. Additionally, contrast echocardiography can help detect apical thrombus formation, a potential complication in patients with severe LV dysfunction and low-flow states [1, 14].

Speckle-tracking strain imaging provides further insights into the myocardial mechanics of TTS. Studies have shown that global longitudinal strain (GLS) is typically reduced in the apical and midventricular segments, while basal segments remain preserved or even hypercontractile [1, 14]. This strain pattern helps differentiate TTS from AMI and other forms of cardiomyopathy [1, 14]. Furthermore, follow-up echocardiography after 4–8 weeks usually demonstrates complete recovery of LV function, confirming the transient nature of TTS [1, 9].

6.3 Cardiac MRI: Differentiating TTS from myocardial infarction and myocarditis

Cardiac magnetic resonance imaging (CMR) is an invaluable tool in distinguishing TTS from other acute cardiac conditions, such as myocardial infarction and myocarditis [1, 14]. One of the most important CMR findings in TTS is the absence of late gadolinium enhancement (LGE). In contrast, in AMI, LGE follows a subendocardial or transmural pattern corresponding to the affected coronary artery territory, reflecting irreversible myocardial necrosis. Myocarditis, another differential diagnosis, typically exhibits patchy, mid-myocardial, or epicardial LGE, which also differs from the findings in TTS [1, 4]. The absence of LGE in TTS confirms that myocardial damage is not due to infarction but rather due to stress-induced myocardial stunning and microvascular dysfunction [1, 4].

Another key feature of CMR in TTS is the presence of myocardial edema on T2-weighted imaging, which reflects acute myocardial inflammation and stress-related injury rather than ischemic necrosis. This finding supports the notion that TTS is a form of stress cardiomyopathy rather than an ischemic event. Additionally, CMR provides a more detailed assessment of LV function and can identify subtle RV involvement, which occurs in approximately 25% of TTS cases [9, 11, 14].

Follow-up CMR imaging after recovery can be particularly helpful in confirming the diagnosis. In TTS, myocardial function typically returns to normal within weeks to months, and the previously noted wall motion abnormalities resolve completely.

This contrasts with ischemic cardiomyopathy, where functional recovery may be incomplete or delayed [1, 9, 12, 14].

7. Clinical implications of imaging findings

The imaging findings in TTS have significant clinical implications for diagnosis, risk stratification, and management. Acute-phase imaging is essential for confirming the diagnosis, ruling out obstructive coronary artery disease (CAD), and identifying complications such as LV thrombus formation, LVOT obstruction, or cardiogenic shock. Follow-up imaging is equally important, as it helps document recovery of LV function, which is a defining feature of TTS and differentiates it from other cardiomyopathies.

Overall, echocardiography provides a rapid, bedside assessment of LV function, making it the first choice in acute settings, while CMR offers superior tissue characterization, helping to rule out AMI and myocarditis. The integration of these imaging modalities allows for a comprehensive evaluation of TTS, ensuring accurate diagnosis and appropriate management.

8. Coronary angiography

Coronary angiography is the gold standard for ruling out obstructive coronary artery disease. It is typically performed in patients presenting with acute chest pain and elevated cardiac biomarkers to exclude myocardial infarction.

9. Indications for coronary angiography in Takotsubo cardiomyopathy

All patients presenting with suspected ACS, including those ultimately diagnosed with TTC, should undergo urgent coronary angiography unless contraindicated. This recommendation follows from the necessity of excluding a true obstructive culprit lesion, which could require revascularization *via* percutaneous coronary intervention (PCI). The primary goal of angiography in TTC is to identify whether acute myocardial ischemia from an epicardial coronary occlusion is responsible for the patient's symptoms and findings. Since the pathophysiology of TTC is distinct from classic atherosclerotic disease, angiography serves as a key differentiator by revealing a lack of obstructive CAD despite significant left ventricular dysfunction.

10. Typical angiographic findings in Takotsubo cardiomyopathy

Most patients with TTC demonstrate normal coronary arteries on angiography, with no evidence of significant luminal stenosis, plaque rupture, or thrombus formation [1, 4]. Studies suggest that approximately 85% of patients with TTC have completely normal coronary arteries, while another 10–15% may exhibit minor luminal irregularities that are not flow-limiting [1, 11, 14]. This pattern contrasts sharply with STEMI, where a culprit lesion with acute thrombosis is usually identified in a major epicardial artery.

A small proportion of patients diagnosed with TTC may have coexisting CAD, raising diagnostic uncertainty [9]. If significant stenosis (≥50% luminal narrowing) is observed, it becomes essential to assess whether this lesion could explain the regional wall motion abnormalities seen on imaging [9, 14]. In cases where the distribution of myocardial dysfunction does not correspond to a single coronary territory, TTC remains a strong consideration. Additionally, TTC typically presents with circumferential myocardial dysfunction, particularly affecting the apical and midventricular segments, whereas ischemic injury due to CAD follows a segmental pattern based on the affected coronary artery.

11. Distinguishing TTC from ACS on coronary angiography

Differentiating TTC from true myocardial infarction on angiography requires a systematic approach. The following key features can help distinguish TTC from ACS:

1. Absence of a culprit lesion—Unlike ACS, where plaque rupture and thrombus formation are expected in a major coronary artery, TTC is characterized by an absence of obstructive disease [14].

2. Non-territorial wall motion abnormalities—In TTC, left ventricular dysfunction does not adhere to a single coronary distribution. Instead, a pattern of apical ballooning with basal hyperkinesis, or alternative variants such as midventricular or basal Takotsubo, is observed [1].

3. Microvascular dysfunction hypothesis—Some theories suggest that TTC results from transient dysfunction at the level of the coronary microcirculation rather than epicardial artery obstruction. This dysfunction is not directly visualized on conventional coronary angiography but can be assessed using invasive microvascular function testing, such as coronary flow reserve (CFR) or the index of microcirculatory resistance (IMR) [4, 9, 11].

While standard coronary angiography can rule out epicardial CAD, it does not provide insight into possible microvascular dysfunction or vasospasm, which have been implicated in TTC pathophysiology. Additional functional testing may be warranted in selected cases where the diagnosis remains uncertain.

12. Advanced coronary imaging and functional testing

In patients with TTC who exhibit borderline or ambiguous coronary findings, advanced imaging techniques such as intravascular ultrasound (IVUS) or optical coherence tomography (OCT) may be utilized. These modalities allow for a detailed assessment of plaque characteristics, helping to exclude subtle atherosclerotic changes or erosions that may have been overlooked in conventional angiography [9, 11].

Another useful tool is fractional flow reserve (FFR), which helps determine whether an intermediate coronary stenosis is functionally significant. If an FFR measurement confirms that a stenosis is not hemodynamically significant, the likelihood of true ACS diminishes, and the diagnosis of TTC becomes more probable [4, 9].

Furthermore, for patients in whom microvascular dysfunction is suspected, coronary vasoreactivity testing using acetylcholine provocation may be performed to assess for endothelial dysfunction and coronary spasm [1, 4, 14]. These additional diagnostic modalities may be particularly useful in cases where recurrent episodes of TTC or persistent myocardial dysfunction are observed.

13. Coexistence of CAD and Takotsubo cardiomyopathy

Although TTC is classically described in patients without significant CAD, there are cases where TTC and obstructive CAD coexist. This presents a diagnostic challenge because wall motion abnormalities in TTC may overlap with those caused by ischemic injury. Clinicians must carefully evaluate whether the regional myocardial dysfunction can be fully explained by the observed coronary lesions or if the pattern of dysfunction suggests an alternative mechanism.

In patients with both CAD and TTC, management should be individualized. If a significant coronary stenosis is present and there is concern for concurrent ACS, PCI may still be warranted. However, unnecessary interventions should be avoided in cases where TTC remains the more likely diagnosis. Cardiac MRI can provide further clarity in such cases by distinguishing between infarct-related injury (which typically shows late gadolinium enhancement in a vascular distribution) and TTC (which lacks LGE or exhibits a diffuse pattern).

14. Clinical implications of coronary angiographic findings

The angiographic findings in TTC have important clinical implications for patient management. The absence of obstructive CAD confirms the diagnosis and prevents unnecessary revascularization procedures, allowing clinicians to focus on supportive therapies. Importantly, coronary angiography also helps identify atypical or secondary forms of Takotsubo syndrome, such as those occurring in pheochromocytoma, subarachnoid hemorrhage, or sepsis-related cardiomyopathy, where similar LV dysfunction patterns may be seen.

Additionally, the angiographic findings influence prognostic considerations. While TTC generally carries a favorable prognosis, patients with preexisting CAD may be at increased risk for cardiovascular events due to underlying atherosclerosis [9, 14]. Consequently, these patients should continue appropriate secondary prevention therapies, including statins, antiplatelet agents, and risk factor modification.

15. Computed tomography (CT) angiography

Computed tomography (CT) angiography serves as a non-invasive alternative to coronary angiography in select cases of Takotsubo cardiomyopathy (TTC), particularly for ruling out obstructive coronary artery disease (CAD) in low-to-intermediate risk patients or those with contraindications to invasive procedures [1, 4, 11]. It provides high-resolution imaging to assess coronary anatomy, left ventricular (LV) function, and regional wall motion abnormalities, aiding in differentiating TTC from acute coronary syndrome (ACS), myocarditis, or other structural heart diseases [14]. Additionally, CT perfusion imaging can evaluate microvascular dysfunction, while delayed contrast-enhanced CT helps detect apical thrombus formation in severe LV dysfunction cases [1, 14]. Though not a replacement for invasive angiography in high-risk patients, CT angiography plays an important role in diagnosis, risk stratification, and follow-up imaging in TTC.

16. Differential diagnosis of Takotsubo cardiomyopathy

Since the clinical presentation overlaps with various cardiac and non-cardiac conditions, it is imperative to consider a broad differential diagnosis to avoid misdiagnosis and ensure appropriate management.

17. Acute coronary syndrome (ACS)

Among the differential diagnoses, ACS, including myocardial infarction (MI), is the most critical condition to rule out. Both ACS and TTC present with chest pain, ST-segment changes on electrocardiography (ECG), and elevated cardiac biomarkers making them nearly indistinguishable based on initial evaluation [1].

The key differentiating factor between ACS and TTC is the coronary angiographic findings. In ACS, a culprit lesion such as an acute thrombus due to plaque rupture or erosion is typically identified in a major epicardial coronary artery [4]. In contrast, TTC is characterized by non-obstructive coronary arteries or only mild luminal irregularities, which cannot explain the extent of myocardial dysfunction observed on imaging [9].

Furthermore, while ACS follows a territorial pattern of myocardial injury, corresponding to the affected coronary artery, TTC manifests as circumferential dysfunction, commonly involving the apical and midventricular segments (though atypical variants exist) [6]. Cardiac MRI can provide additional differentiation by showing late gadolinium enhancement (LGE) in ischemic infarcts, whereas TTC typically lacks LGE, indicating the absence of irreversible myocardial damage [9, 14].

Despite these distinctions, differentiating TTC from ACS remains a challenge in the acute setting, emphasizing the need for early coronary angiography to confirm the diagnosis.

18. Myocarditis

Myocarditis is an inflammatory condition of the myocardium that can closely mimic TTC, presenting with chest pain, ECG abnormalities, and elevated cardiac biomarkers. Viral myocarditis, in particular, is a frequent consideration in patients presenting with symptoms suggestive of myocardial ischemia but without obstructive CAD [9].

A crucial differentiator between myocarditis and TTC is cardiac magnetic resonance imaging (MRI). In myocarditis, late gadolinium enhancement (LGE) is typically present, often in a non-ischemic pattern (such as the mid-myocardial or subepicardial layers), reflecting areas of myocardial inflammation or fibrosis. In contrast, TTC usually lacks LGE, indicating transient rather than permanent myocardial injury [6, 9].

Additionally, myocarditis may be accompanied by systemic inflammatory markers, such as elevated C-reactive protein (CRP) and erythrocyte sedimentation rate

(ESR), and may be associated with a recent viral illness. Endomyocardial biopsy may be necessary in selected cases where myocarditis remains a diagnostic concern [6].

19. Pheochromocytoma-induced cardiomyopathy

Pheochromocytoma, a catecholamine-secreting tumor of the adrenal medulla, can cause a clinical syndrome similar to TTC. The excessive secretion of epinephrine and norepinephrine in pheochromocytoma results in severe vasoconstriction, increased myocardial oxygen demand, and direct myocardial toxicity, leading to reversible LV dysfunction, often resembling TTC [6].

Unlike classic TTC, which is typically triggered by emotional or physical stress, pheochromocytoma-induced cardiomyopathy may occur spontaneously or in association with paroxysmal hypertensive crises. These patients frequently exhibit severe hypertension, tachycardia, headaches, diaphoresis, and palpitations, raising suspicion for an underlying neuroendocrine disorder [6].

Diagnosis requires biochemical testing, including plasma-free metanephrines or 24-hour urinary metanephrines, which have high sensitivity and specificity for pheochromocytoma. CT or MRI of the adrenal glands is then performed to localize the tumor [11]. Treatment involves surgical resection of the tumor, with preoperative alpha-adrenergic blockade to prevent hypertensive crises [11].

20. Pulmonary embolism (PE)

Pulmonary embolism is a life-threatening condition that can present with chest pain, dyspnea, and ECG abnormalities, making it a crucial differential diagnosis in patients suspected of TTC. In some cases, right ventricular strain due to a large PE can lead to reversible right ventricular dysfunction, mimicking the acute heart failure seen in TTC.

A key distinction is that PE is more likely to be associated with:

- Evidence of right heart strain on echocardiography (e.g., right ventricular dilation and McConnell's sign) [9].

- CT pulmonary angiography (CTPA) confirming the presence of pulmonary emboli [14].

Given the potential for sudden hemodynamic deterioration, clinicians should have a low threshold for performing CTPA in patients with unexplained dyspnea, tachycardia, or risk factors for venous thromboembolism.

21. Other cardiomyopathies

Several other forms of cardiomyopathy should be considered in the differential diagnosis of TTC, including:

1. Hypertrophic cardiomyopathy (HCM)—Characterized by asymmetric left ventricular hypertrophy, often involving the septum, with or without left ventricular outflow tract (LVOT) obstruction. Genetic testing may be indicated in familial cases [6].

2. Dilated cardiomyopathy (DCM)—Presents with global systolic dysfunction and chamber dilation, distinguishing it from the transient regional dysfunction seen in TTC [6].

3. Left ventricular noncompaction cardiomyopathy (LVNC)—A rare entity with excessive trabeculations and deep recesses seen on echocardiography or MRI [9, 14].

This table provides a structured comparison of key diagnostic findings across these conditions, focusing on wall motion abnormalities, coronary angiography, echocardiographic patterns, cardiac MRI characteristics, and ECG changes. The distinctions highlighted help differentiate Takotsubo cardiomyopathy from ischemic and non-ischemic myocardial syndromes, aiding in accurate diagnosis and clinical decision-making.

Table 1 provides a structured comparison of key diagnostic findings across these conditions, focusing on wall motion abnormalities, coronary angiography, echocardiographic patterns, cardiac MRI characteristics, and ECG changes. The distinctions highlighted help differentiate Takotsubo cardiomyopathy from ischemic and non-ischemic myocardial syndromes, aiding in accurate diagnosis and clinical decision-making.

Feature	Takotsubo cardiomyopathy (TTC)	Acute coronary syndrome (ACS)	Myocarditis	Pheochromocy toma-induced cardiomyopathy
Regional wall motion abnormalities (RWMA)	Apical and midventricular ballooning with basal hyperkinesis (does NOT follow a coronary territory)	Follows a specific coronary artery distribution	Patchy, non-territorial involvement	Diffuse or mid-basal involvement (can resemble TTC)
Left ventricular function	Transient severe dysfunction recovers within weeks	LV dysfunction dependent on infarct size, often permanent	Variable may lead to long-term dysfunction	Severe LV dysfunction, often with hypertensive crisis
Coronary angiography	No obstructive coronary artery disease	Obstructive coronary artery disease (culprit lesion in ACS)	No significant CAD	No significant CAD, but vasospasm possible
Echocardiography	Apical ballooning, hypercontractile basal segments, ± LVOT obstruction	Regional wall motion abnormalities in a vascular distribution	Diffuse hypokinesis or focal involvement	Hypercontractility of basal LV, ± LVOT obstruction
Speckle-tracking strain imaging	Apical strain severely reduced, basal strain preserved or increased	Reduced strain corresponding to infarcted area	Global strain reduction with non-territorial distribution	Global or mid-basal strain reduction
Cardiac MRI: late gadolinium enhancement (LGE)	Absent (no myocardial necrosis)	Present in subendocardial or transmural infarcted areas	Present in a patchy, mid-myocardial or epicardial pattern	Absent or mild, unless ischemic damage occurs

Feature	Takotsubo cardiomyopathy (TTC)	Acute coronary syndrome (ACS)	Myocarditis	Pheochromocytoma-induced cardiomyopathy
Cardiac MRI: T2-weighted imaging (edema assessment)	Myocardial edema in affected segments	Edema in infarcted area	Diffuse or patchy myocardial edema	Diffuse myocardial edema from catecholamine toxicity
QT interval (ECG)	Prolonged QT interval, deep T-wave inversions in recovery phase	ST-segment changes (ST-elevation in STEMI, ST-depression in NSTEMI)	Diffuse ST changes, PR depression possible	Prolonged QT, possible tachyarrhythmias
Recovery timeline	LV function normalizes in 1–4 weeks	Permanent damage possible if infarction is large	Variable recovery may develop chronic heart failure	Reversible with tumor removal, but severe cases can lead to chronic cardiomyopathy

Table 1.
Comparative features of Takotsubo cardiomyopathy, acute coronary syndrome, myocarditis, and pheochromocytoma-induced cardiomyopathy.

22. Acute management

22.1 Supportive care

- Hospitalization and monitoring: Most patients with TTC require admission to a coronary care unit (CCU) for continuous monitoring due to the risk of arrhythmias, cardiogenic shock, or thromboembolic complications [1].

- Oxygen therapy: If oxygen saturation is low or there is respiratory distress, supplemental oxygen is administered to improve myocardial oxygenation [14].

- Pain relief: Chest pain, often mimicking myocardial infarction (MI), is treated with analgesics, avoiding nonsteroidal anti-inflammatory drugs (NSAIDs) due to their potential adverse cardiovascular effects [1].

22.2 Heart failure management

- Diuretics: Used in fluid-overloaded patients to relieve symptoms of pulmonary congestion and edema. However, careful titration is needed, as excessive diuresis can lead to hypotension, particularly in those with left ventricular outflow tract (LVOT) obstruction [14].

- ACE inhibitors/ARBs: Angiotensin-converting enzyme inhibitors (ACEIs) or angiotensin receptor blockers (ARBs) may be initiated in cases of persistent LV dysfunction to improve ventricular remodeling and reduce afterload [11].

- Beta-blockers: Typically avoided in the acute phase, especially in patients with LVOT obstruction, as they may exacerbate hemodynamic instability [14].

22.3 Anticoagulation and thromboembolism prevention

- Risk of left ventricular (LV) thrombosis: Due to severe LV dysfunction and akinesis, some TTC patients develop apical thrombus, which increases the risk of systemic embolization (e.g., stroke and limb ischemia) [11].
- Anticoagulation therapy:
  - o Short-term anticoagulation (e.g., warfarin and direct oral anticoagulants [DOACs]) is recommended in patients with severe LV dysfunction (LVEF <30%) or documented LV thrombus [1].
  - o Prophylactic anticoagulation may be considered in patients at high risk for thromboembolism [11].

23. Long-term management

23.1 Beta-blockers for prevention

- While beta-blockers have not consistently shown to prevent recurrence, they may be beneficial for:
  - o Reducing catecholamine surges, which are thought to contribute to TTC pathophysiology [6].
  - o Managing arrhythmias and hypertension in patients with persistent cardiovascular risk factors [6].
  - o Patients with concurrent heart failure or arrhythmias should remain on beta-blockers long-term [6].

23.2 Lifestyle modifications

Since emotional and physical stressors trigger ~67% of TTC cases, stress management strategies are crucial for recurrence prevention [11]. Recommended interventions include:

- Mindfulness meditation and cognitive-behavioral therapy (CBT): Helps reduce anxiety and emotional stress that may precipitate TTC.
- Regular physical activity: Low- to moderate-intensity exercise (e.g., walking, yoga, and tai chi) promotes cardiovascular health while reducing stress levels.
- Avoiding catecholamine surges: Avoidance of excessive caffeine, stimulants, or abrupt discontinuation of medications (e.g., beta-blockers) is important.

23.3 Psychological support and mental health care

- Emotional stress as a trigger: Many TTC patients experience major emotional distress (e.g., grief, anxiety, and depression), warranting psychiatric or psychological evaluation.

- Counseling and support groups: Programs such as stress management workshops, therapy groups, and cognitive therapy may improve coping mechanisms and reduce recurrence risk.

- Screening for depression and anxiety: Patients with TTC should undergo screening for depression and post-traumatic stress disorder (PTSD), particularly those with prior psychiatric disorders.

23.4 Follow-up care and monitoring

- Cardiology follow-up: Regular follow-ups with echocardiography are crucial to monitor left ventricular function recovery (which usually occurs within 1–4 weeks but may take months in some cases).

- Electrocardiographic monitoring: Persistent QT prolongation may predispose to arrhythmias, necessitating serial ECGs.

- Monitoring for recurrence: While rare (~1.8% per patient-year), recurrences may occur, particularly in older patients or those with underlying hypertension, diabetes, or pulmonary disease [1].

24. Recurrence and long-term considerations

Although TTC is often self-limiting and left ventricular function normalizes within weeks to months, recurrence remains a concern in high-risk patients [1].

24.1 Factors associated with higher recurrence risk

- Older age and male gender: While TTC predominantly affects postmenopausal women, older men who develop TTC tend to have a higher risk of recurrence and complications [1, 2].

- Comorbid conditions: Chronic conditions such as diabetes, pulmonary disease, and prior cardiovascular disease increase the risk of recurrent episodes [6].

- Severe emotional or physical stressors: Patients with frequent emotional distress, anxiety, or PTSD are more prone to recurrence [5].

24.2 Long-term complications and monitoring

- Heart failure: While rare, some TTC patients experience persistent LV dysfunction, requiring long-term heart failure management [12].

- Arrhythmias: Prolonged QT intervals and repolarization abnormalities can increase the risk of ventricular arrhythmias and sudden cardiac events [1].

- Psychosocial impact: Many TTC patients experience anxiety or PTSD after their initial event, necessitating long-term psychological support [1].

24.3 Medication adherence

- Patients should be encouraged to adhere to prescribed medications such as beta-blockers, ACE inhibitors, or anticoagulants (if indicated) to reduce recurrence risk and complications [6].

- Discontinuation of medications, particularly beta-blockers or antihypertensives, should be done cautiously under medical supervision [1].

25. Future directions and research

Ongoing research in TTS is focused on improving diagnosis, treatment, and long-term management to reduce recurrence and complications. Advanced cardiac MRI protocols are being explored to provide deeper insights into myocardial changes during acute TTS episodes, helping differentiate it from other cardiomyopathies. There is a growing need for evidence-based treatment guidelines, as clinical trials are evaluating the efficacy of pharmacological therapies (e.g., beta-blockers, ACE inhibitors, and anticoagulants) and non-pharmacological interventions such as stress reduction techniques and lifestyle modifications. Long-term management strategies are being studied to determine how psychological support and autonomic regulation can mitigate recurrence risk. Additionally, research is focusing on identifying recurrence predictors, with a particular emphasis on whether beta-blockers or other medications can effectively prevent future TTS episodes. As understanding of TTS evolves, these advancements will help refine personalized treatment strategies and improve patient outcomes.

26. Conclusion

TTC has redefined the interplay between emotional stress and cardiac dysfunction, revealing a dynamic neurocardiac interface. Once considered benign, TTC now warrants recognition as a complex syndrome with acute and chronic risks, including heart failure, arrhythmias, and recurrence.

Innovations in cardiac imaging and emerging biomarkers have enhanced diagnostic precision, yet treatment remains largely supportive. The central roles of catecholaminergic surge and microvascular dysfunction emphasize the need for integrative, multidisciplinary care encompassing cardiovascular, neuropsychiatric, and psychosocial domains.

Future priorities include randomized trials and mechanistic studies to clarify pathogenesis, guide tailored therapies, and reduce recurrence. TTC stands as a model of mind-heart interaction, underscoring the imperative for holistic, patient-centered cardiology.

Author details

Andrew Ndakotsu
MedStar Health, Baltimore, Maryland, USA

*Address all correspondence to: ninoskills@gmail.com

References

[1] Templin C, Ghadri JR, Diekmann J, et al. Clinical features and outcomes of Takotsubo (stress) cardiomyopathy. The New England Journal of Medicine. 2015;**373**(10):929-938. DOI: 10.1056/NEJMoa1406761

[2] Sykes R, Ang DTY, Berry C. Takotsubo is an acute myocardial ischaemic syndrome. European Heart Journal. 2025;**46**(17):1582-1585. DOI: 10.1093/eurheartj/ehaf020

[3] Tofield A. Hikaru Sato and Takotsubo cardiomyopathy. European Heart Journal. 2016;**37**(37):2812. DOI: 10.1093/eurheartj/ehw367

[4] Akashi YJ, Goldstein DS, Barbaro G, Ueyama T. Takotsubo cardiomyopathy: A new form of acute, reversible heart failure. Circulation. 2008;**118**(25): 2754-2762. DOI: 10.1161/CIRCULATIONAHA.108.767012

[5] Chan C, Elliott J, Troughton R, et al. Acute myocardial infarction and stress cardiomyopathy following the Christchurch earthquakes. PLoS One. 2013;**8**(7):e68504. DOI: 10.1371/journal.pone.0068504

[6] Singh T, Khan H, Gamble DT, Scally C, Newby DE, Dawson D. Takotsubo syndrome: Pathophysiology, emerging concepts, and clinical implications. Circulation. 2022;**145**(13):1002-1019. DOI: 10.1161/CIRCULATIONAHA.121.055854. Epub 2022 Mar 28. Erratum in: Circulation. 2022;**145**(20):e1053. DOI: 10.1161/CIR.0000000000001075

[7] Deshmukh A, Kumar G, Pant S, Rihal C, Murugiah K, Mehta JL. Prevalence of Takotsubo cardiomyopathy in the United States. American Heart Journal. 2012;**164**(1):66-71.e1. DOI: 10.1016/j.ahj.2012.03.020

[8] Khera R, Light-McGroary K, Zahr F, Horwitz PA, Girotra S. Trends in hospitalization for takotsubo cardiomyopathy in the United States. American Heart Journal. 2016;**172**:53-63. DOI: 10.1016/j.ahj.2015.10.022. Epub 2015 Nov 14

[9] Bossone E, Lyon A, Citro R, et al. Takotsubo cardiomyopathy: An integrated multi-imaging approach. European Heart Journal Cardiovascular Imaging. 2014;**15**(4):366-377. DOI: 10.1093/ehjci/jet167

[10] Assad J, Femia G, Pender P, Badie T, Rajaratnam R. Takotsubo syndrome: A review of presentation, diagnosis and management. Clinical Medicine Insights: Cardiology. 2022;(16):11795468211065782. DOI: 10.1177/11795468211065782

[11] Pelliccia F, Kaski JC, Crea F, Camici PG. Pathophysiology of Takotsubo syndrome. Circulation. 2017;**135**(24):2426-2441. DOI: 10.1161/CIRCULATIONAHA.116.027121

[12] Kurisu S, Kihara Y. Tako-tsubo cardiomyopathy: Clinical presentation and underlying mechanism. Journal of Cardiology. 2012;**60**(6):429-437. DOI: 10.1016/j.jjcc.2012.06.015. Epub 2012 Oct 15

[13] Boyd B, Solh T. Takotsubo cardiomyopathy: Review of broken heart syndrome. JAAPA. 2020;**33**(3):24-29. DOI: 10.1097/01.JAA.0000654368.35241.fc

[14] Ghadri JR, Wittstein IS, Prasad A, Sharkey S, Dote K, Akashi YJ, et al.

International expert consensus document on Takotsubo syndrome (part I): Clinical characteristics, diagnostic criteria, and pathophysiology. European Heart Journal. 2018;**39**(22):2032-2046. DOI: 10.1093/eurheartj/ehy076

Chapter 4

Aortic Stenosis

Sultan Alotaibi

Abstract

Aortic stenosis (AS) is the most common valvular heart disease in developed nations and a major cause of morbidity and mortality in older adults. Progressive narrowing of the aortic valve leads to left ventricular outflow obstruction, hypertrophy, and eventual heart failure. This chapter reviews AS pathophysiology, clinical assessment, and contemporary management, emphasizing timely diagnosis and intervention. Echocardiography is the diagnostic cornerstone, with advanced imaging and biomarkers aiding in complex cases. Surgical aortic valve replacement (SAVR) remains standard for low-risk patients, while transcatheter aortic valve replacement (TAVR) now offers comparable outcomes across all risk categories. No medical therapy alters disease progression; management focuses on symptom monitoring, comorbidity control, and appropriate procedural referral. Future directions include enhanced valve durability, expanded minimally invasive options, and AI-driven personalized care.

Keywords: aortic valve stenosis, echocardiography, doppler, transcatheter aortic valve replacement, aortic valve/surgery, heart valve prosthesis implantation, left ventricular hypertrophy, cardiac imaging techniques, heart team, cardiac catheterization

1. Introduction

Aortic stenosis (AS) is the most prevalent valvular heart disease in developed countries, accounting for significant morbidity and mortality, especially in older adults. It is characterized by progressive narrowing of the aortic valve orifice, leading to obstruction of left ventricular outflow and subsequent pressure overload. This increased afterload results in compensatory left ventricular hypertrophy, diastolic dysfunction, and ultimately heart failure if untreated. The natural history of AS involves a prolonged asymptomatic phase, followed by symptom onset which heralds a poor prognosis. Early identification and timely intervention are therefore essential to improve patient outcomes. Advances in diagnostic modalities, surgical techniques, and transcatheter therapies have revolutionized management, offering individualized treatment options based on patient risk profiles and preferences [1, 2].

Of note, AS does not exist in isolation but often overlaps with various forms of cardiomyopathy. The chronic pressure overload from AS leads to left ventricular hypertrophy, impaired relaxation, and eventually a restrictive physiology that resembles hypertrophic cardiomyopathy in some patients. Conversely, patients with pre-existing cardiomyopathies, such as hypertrophic obstructive cardiomyopathy, dilated cardiomyopathy, or infiltrative types, may have more complex hemodynamics

IntechOpen

and poorer outcomes when AS develops. This interaction underscores the importance of distinguishing primary myocardial disease from secondary changes due to valvular obstruction [3, 4].

2. Clinical evaluation and diagnosis

The clinical assessment of AS starts with a thorough history and physical examination. Classic symptoms include exertional dyspnea, angina, and syncope, reflecting significant hemodynamic compromise. However, symptoms can be subtle or absent in early disease stages, emphasizing the need for vigilance. Auscultation may reveal a harsh, crescendo-decrescendo systolic murmur best heard at the right upper sternal border with radiation to the carotids, diminished second heart sound, and delayed carotid upstroke (parvus et tardus) [5]. Nevertheless, clinical examination alone lacks sensitivity, and echocardiography remains indispensable.

Transthoracic echocardiography (TTE) is the gold standard for diagnosis and quantification of AS severity (92% sensitivity and 96% specificity). Key parameters include peak aortic jet velocity, mean transvalvular gradient, and aortic valve area (AVA) calculated using the continuity equation. Severe AS is defined by a peak velocity $\geq$ 4.0 m/s, mean gradient $\geq$40 mm Hg, or AVA <1.0 cm^2. in the latest guidelines, advanced imaging modalities (3D echocardiography), cardiac computed tomography (CT), cardiac magnetic resonance imaging (MRI) are given greater importance, especially in discordant cases, for more precise diagnosis [6].

Low-flow, low-gradient AS, particularly in patients with reduced left ventricular ejection fraction (LVEF), poses diagnostic challenges. Dobutamine stress echocardiography helps distinguish true severe AS from pseudo-severe forms by assessing contractile reserve and changes in gradients [7]. Recent registry and guideline updates suggest that a lack of contractile reserve should not necessarily exclude intervention, especially when CT calcium scoring strongly supports severe AS [6].

Cardiac CT calcium scoring provides quantitative assessment of valvular calcification, with sex-specific Agatston thresholds aiding in diagnosis and prognosis [8]. Cardiac MRI complements evaluation by assessing ventricular volumes, function, and myocardial fibrosis, which has prognostic significance [9].

Exercise testing can unmask symptoms and assess functional capacity in asymptomatic patients, guiding timing of intervention [10]. Biomarkers, such as B-type natriuretic peptide (BNP), correlate with disease severity and outcomes but are not

Left ventricular pattern	Aortic stenosis (AS)	Cardiomyopathies
Concentric hypertrophy	Classic in severe AS	Less common (can mimic hypertrophic cardiomyopathy)
Asymmetric septal hypertrophy	Rare, except overlap with cardiomyopathy	Hallmark of hypertrophic cardiomyopathy
Dilated left ventricle with low ejection fraction	Late/end-stage AS	Dilated cardiomyopathy
Restrictive physiology	Rare in pure AS	Restrictive/infiltrative cardiomyopathies (amyloid, Fabry, sarcoid)

Table 1.
Types of left ventricular remodeling in aortic stenosis versus cardiomyopathies.

	Aortic stenosis (AS) alone	Coexistent cardiomyopathy
Symptoms	Typical triad (angina, syncope, dyspnea)	Disproportionate heart failure symptoms
Echocardiography	Concentric left ventricular hypertrophy, high gradient	Asymmetric septal hypertrophy, apical thickening, restrictive filling
Cardiac MRI	Mid-wall fibrosis	Diffuse fibrosis, infiltration, amyloid pattern
Biomarkers	BNP proportional to AS severity	BNP disproportionately elevated

Table 2.
Clinical and imaging red flags in aortic stenosis with possible cardiomyopathy.

diagnostic on their own [11]. Invasive hemodynamic assessment *via* cardiac catheterization is reserved for cases with discordant noninvasive findings or when coronary angiography to exclude obstructive disease is indicated [12].

Importantly, differentiation between AS-induced left ventricular hypertrophy and coexistent cardiomyopathy is essential (**Tables 1** and **2**). Echocardiographic strain imaging and cardiac MRI help identify diffuse fibrosis, infiltration, or phenotypes consistent with hypertrophic or restrictive cardiomyopathy, which may change prognosis and influence timing of intervention [13].

3. Timing of intervention

The timing of aortic valve replacement (AVR) is critical due to the poor prognosis of symptomatic severe AS, which carries a high mortality risk within 2 to 5 years if untreated [14]. Guidelines from the American College of Cardiology/American Heart Association (ACC/AHA) and European Society of Cardiology/European Association for Cardio-Thoracic Surgery (ESC/EACTS) recommend AVR for all patients with symptomatic severe AS regardless of surgical risk [6, 15].

In asymptomatic patients, indications for AVR include left ventricular systolic dysfunction (LVEF <50%), very severe AS (peak velocity ≥ 5.0 m/s), rapid disease progression (>0.3 m/s per year), abnormal exercise test findings (symptoms or hypotension), and markedly elevated BNP levels [10]. AVR is considered a Class IIa alternative (rather than only observation) in asymptomatic severe AS with high-risk features and preserved LVEF if procedural risk is low [6]. Patients with low-flow, low-gradient AS and reduced LVEF require careful evaluation with dobutamine stress echocardiography or CT calcium scoring to confirm severity [7]. Decision-making must now more explicitly incorporate the patient's lifetime trajectory, Heart Valve Centre expertise, and shared decision-making [16].

Multidisciplinary heart team discussion is essential to tailor intervention timing based on risks, comorbidities, and patient preferences [15]. Emerging evidence suggests potential benefits of earlier intervention even in select asymptomatic patients, though more data are needed to refine guidelines [17].

4. Medical management

Currently, no pharmacologic therapies have been proven to modify the course of AS. Management focuses on symptom relief and treatment of comorbidities such as hypertension and heart failure [18]. Clinical trials investigating statins and renin-angiotensin system inhibitors have failed to demonstrate significant impact on valve progression [19, 20]. Vasodilators should be used cautiously due to the fixed obstruction and risk of hypotension, while diuretics may be employed judiciously to control volume overload [6].

In patients with AS and coexisting cardiomyopathy phenotypes (e.g., ATTR amyloidosis), the interplay of medical therapies targeting the myocardial disease should be considered in addition to standard valvular care [21].

Regular monitoring with clinical and echocardiographic follow-up is essential to detect symptom onset or ventricular dysfunction that prompt intervention [6, 15]. Follow-up should now more frequently incorporate imaging markers (e.g. LV strain, fibrosis) and biomarker trends to anticipate decompensation earlier [6].

5. Surgical aortic valve replacement (SAVR)

SAVR continues to be the standard therapy for eligible patients with severe AS, especially younger individuals and those with low to intermediate surgical risk [6]. The procedure involves excision of the diseased valve and implantation of either a mechanical or bioprosthetic valve. Mechanical valves provide excellent durability but necessitate lifelong anticoagulation, increasing bleeding risk [22]. Bioprosthetic valves avoid chronic anticoagulation but have limited longevity due to structural valve degeneration, particularly in younger patients [23]. Advances in surgical techniques and perioperative care have reduced operative mortality to less than 2% in low-risk cohorts [24].

Patient selection incorporates surgical risk scores such as the Society of Thoracic Surgeons (STS) risk score or EuroSCORE II, alongside assessment of frailty and comorbidities [24]. Indications include symptomatic severe AS, asymptomatic severe AS with LV dysfunction, and selected cases with very severe or rapidly progressive disease [6, 15]; lifetime planning (e.g. future redo, valve-in-valve) is emphasized when choosing prosthesis type and surgical strategy [6]. SAVR may also be combined with coronary artery bypass grafting when indicated [25]. The latest also suggest increased use of coronary CT angiography preoperatively in selected patients with low pretest probability of coronary artery disease [6].

6. Transcatheter aortic valve replacement (TAVR)

TAVR has transformed AS treatment, initially reserved for patients at prohibitive or high surgical risk, now expanded to intermediate and low-risk patients based on robust randomized trials [26–28]. The procedure involves percutaneous implantation of a bioprosthetic valve via transfemoral or alternative access routes. Imaging with CT is crucial for procedural planning, including annulus sizing and vascular access assessment [29]. Devices include balloon-expandable and self-expanding valves, each with distinct profiles and complication risks [30, 31].

Complications include paravalvular leak, vascular injury, conduction disturbances necessitating pacemaker implantation, and stroke [32]. Recent studies demonstrate comparable or superior outcomes of TAVR versus SAVR in selected patients, with shorter recovery times [33, 34]. The heart team approach is essential for optimal patient selection and management [6].

7. Post-procedural care and follow-up

After aortic valve replacement, patients require careful monitoring for complications, such as prosthetic valve dysfunction, endocarditis, and thromboembolism. Regular echocardiographic surveillance assesses valve function and ventricular remodeling. Antithrombotic therapy post-AVR is individualized based on valve type, comorbidities, and bleeding risk. Cardiac rehabilitation and lifestyle modifications improve functional status and quality of life [6].

8. Future directions and emerging technologies

Future research focuses on improving valve durability, reducing thrombogenicity, and expanding valve-in-valve and valve-in-TAVR procedures. Novel valve materials and designs aim to enhance longevity and biocompatibility. Pharmacologic agents targeting calcification pathways and inflammatory processes are under investigation [16, 35]. Advances in artificial intelligence promise enhanced imaging analysis and personalized risk prediction [36]. Expanding access to care and managing the growing AS population remain challenges globally [37].

9. Conclusion

AS is a common and serious valvular disease with evolving management strategies. Timely diagnosis, accurate severity assessment, and individualized treatment involving surgical or transcatheter interventions are critical to improving outcomes. Ongoing advances in valve technology and medical therapies hold promise for further progress in this field.

Another evolving area is the intersection between AS and cardiomyopathies. Recognition of myocardial disease beyond valvular obstruction is increasingly important, since coexistent hypertrophic, restrictive, or dilated phenotypes can influence patient symptoms, LV remodeling after valve replacement, and long-term survival.

Author details

Sultan Alotaibi
Cardiac Center, King Fahad Armed Forces Hospital, Jeddah, Saudi Arabia

*Address all correspondence to: sultan.otb@gmail.com

References

[1] Rajamannan NM, Evans FJ, Aikawa E. Calcific aortic valve disease: Not simply a degenerative process. Circulation. 2011;**124**(16):1783-1791

[2] Lindman BR, Clavel MA, Mathieu P. Calcific aortic stenosis. Nature Reviews Disease Primers. 2016;**2**:16006

[3] Maron MS, Olivotto I, Zenovich AG, Link MS, Pandian NG, Kuvin JT, et al. Hypertrophic cardiomyopathy is predominantly a disease of left ventricular outflow tract obstruction. Circulation. 2006;**114**(21):2232-2239

[4] Everett Russell J, Treibel Thomas A, Fukui M, Lee H, Rigolli M, Singh A, et al. Extracellular myocardial volume in patients with aortic stenosis. JACC. 2020;**75**(3):304-316

[5] Otto CM. Valvular aortic stenosis: Disease severity and timing of intervention. Journal of the American College of Cardiology. 2006;**47**(11):2141-2151

[6] Praz F, Borger MA, Lanz J, Marin-Cuartas M, Abreu A, Adamo M, et al. ESC/EACTS guidelines for the management of valvular heart disease: Developed by the task force for the management of valvular heart disease of the European Society of Cardiology (ESC) and the European Association for Cardio-Thoracic Surgery (EACTS). European Journal of Cardio-Thoracic Surgery. 2025;**67**(8):ezaf276

[7] Monin JL, Guéret P. [Calcified aortic stenosis with left ventricular dysfunction and low transvalvular gradients. Must one reject surgery in certain cases?]. Archives des Maladies du Coeur et des Vaisseaux. Sep 2003;**96**(9):864-870. PMID: 14571640

[8] Clavel M, Pibarot P, Messika-Zeitoun D, et al. Impact of aortic valve calcification, as measured by MDCT, on survival in patients with aortic stenosis: Results of an international registry study. Journal of the American College of Cardiology. 23 Sep 2014;**64**(12):1202-1213

[9] Dweck MR, Joshi S, Murigu T. Midwall fibrosis is an independent predictor of mortality in patients with aortic stenosis. Journal of the American College of Cardiology. 2011;**58**(12):1271-1279

[10] Magne J, Lancellotti P, Piérard LA. Exercise testing in asymptomatic severe aortic stenosis. JACC: Cardiovascular Imaging. Feb 2014;7(2):188-199

[11] Weber M, Arnold R, Rau M, Brandt R, Berkovitsch A, Mitrovic V, et al. Relation of N-terminal pro–B-type natriuretic peptide to severity of valvular aortic stenosis. The American Journal of Cardiology. 15 Sep 2004;**94**(6):740-745

[12] Saikrishnan N, Kumar G, Sawaya FJ, Lerakis S, Yoganathan AP. Accurate assessment of aortic stenosis: A review of diagnostic modalities and hemodynamics. Circulation. 14 Jan 2014;**129**(2):244-253. Available from: https://www.ahajournals.org/doi/full/10.1161/CIRCULATIONAHA.113.002310

[13] Habib G, Bucciarelli-Ducci C, Caforio ALP, Cardim N, Charron P, Cosyns B, et al. Multimodality Imaging in Restrictive Cardiomyopathies: An EACVI expert consensus document in collaboration with the "Working Group on myocardial and pericardial diseases" of the European Society of

Cardiology Endorsed by The Indian Academy of Echocardiography. European Heart Journal Cardiovascular Imaging. 2017;**18**(10):1090-1121

[14] Ross J Jr, Braunwald E. Aortic stenosis. Circulation. 1968;**38**(1 Suppl): 61-67

[15] Otto CM. 2020 ACC/AHA guideline for the management of patients with valvular heart disease. Circulation. 2021;**143**(5):e72-e227

[16] Kovarovic B, Helbock R, Baylous K, Rotman OM, Slepian MJ, Bluestein D. Visions of TAVR future: Development and optimization of a second generation novel polymeric TAVR. Journal of Biomechanical Engineering. 2022;**144**(6):061008 (pages 1-10)

[17] Kaul S. Aortic valve replacement for asymptomatic severe aortic stenosis: Is enthusiasm exceeding the evidence? Journal of the American College of Cardiology. 2025;**85**(14):1511-1514

[18] Osnabrugge RL, Mylotte D, Head SJ. Aortic stenosis in the elderly. Journal of the American College of Cardiology. 2013;**62**(11):1002-1012

[19] Cowell SJ, Newby DE, Prescott RJ, Bloomfield P, Reid J, Northridge DB, et al. A randomized trial of intensive lipid-lowering therapy in calcific aortic stenosis. New England Journal of Medicine. 9 Jun 2005;**352**(23):2389-2397

[20] Goh SS, Sia CH, Ngiam NJ, Tan BY, Lee PS, Tay EL, et al. Effect of renin-angiotensin blockers on left ventricular remodeling in severe aortic stenosis. The American Journal of Cardiology. 1 Jun 2017;**119**(11):1839-1845

[21] Nitsche C, Dobner S, Rosenblum HR, Patel KP, Longhi S, Yilmaz A, et al. Cardiac transthyretin amyloidosis treatment improves outcomes after aortic valve replacement for severe stenosis. European Heart Journal. 2025;**46**:ehaf362

[22] Head SJ, Çelik M, Kappetein AP. Mechanical versus bioprosthetic aortic valve replacement. European Heart Journal. 2017;**38**(28):2183-2191

[23] Rodriguez-Gabella T, Voisine P, Puri R, Pibarot P, Rodés-Cabau J. Aortic bioprosthetic valve durability. JACC. 2017;**70**(8):1013-1028

[24] Nashef SA, Roques F, Sharples LD, Nilsson J, Smith C, Goldstone AR, et al. EuroSCORE II. European Journal of Cardio-Thoracic Surgery. 2012;**41**(4): 734-744. discussion 44-5

[25] Kobayashi KJ, Williams JA, Nwakanma L, Gott VL, Baumgartner WA, Conte JV. Aortic valve replacement and concomitant coronary artery bypass: Assessing the impact of multiple grafts. The Annals of Thoracic Surgery. 2007;**83**(3):969-978

[26] Leon MB, Smith CR, Mack MJ, Makkar RR, Svensson LG, Kodali SK, et al. Transcatheter or surgical aortic-valve replacement in intermediate-risk patients. New England Journal of Medicine. 2016;**374**(17):1609-1620

[27] Vekstein AM, Wegermann ZK, Manandhar P, Mack MJ, Cohen DJ, Hughes GC, et al. Outcomes of transcatheter aortic valve replacement in low-risk patients in the United States: A report from the STS/ACC TVT registry. Circulation. 2025;**151**(16):1134-1146

[28] Mack Michael J, Leon Martin B, Thourani Vinod H, Pibarot P, Hahn Rebecca T, Genereux P, et al. Transcatheter aortic-valve replacement in low-risk patients at five years. New England Journal of Medicine. 2023;**389**(21):1949-1960

[29] Blanke P, Weir-McCall JR, Achenbach S, Delgado V, Hausleiter J, Jilaihawi H, et al. Computed tomography imaging in the context of transcatheter aortic valve implantation (TAVI)/ transcatheter aortic valve replacement (TAVR): An expert consensus document of the Society of Cardiovascular Computed Tomography. JACC: Cardiovascular Imaging. 2019;**12**(1):1-24

[30] Senguttuvan NB, Bhatt H, Balakrishnan VK, Krishnamoorthy P, Goel S, Reddy PMK, et al. The safety and efficacy of balloon-expandable versus self-expanding trans-catheter aortic valve replacement in high-risk patients with severe symptomatic aortic stenosis. Frontiers in Cardiovascular Medicine. 2023;**10**:1130354

[31] Bihag Z, Patel J, Mather JF, Hagberg R, Haider J, Azemi T, et al. 6 year follow-up of balloon-expandable versus self-expanding transcatheter aortic valves: A propensity-matched analysis. The American Journal of Cardiology. 2025;**253**:78-85

[32] Généreux P, Piazza N, Alu Maria C, Nazif T, Hahn Rebecca T, et al. Valve academic research consortium 3: Updated endpoint definitions for aortic valve clinical research. JACC. 2021;**77**(21):2717-2746

[33] Blankenberg S, Seiffert M, Vonthein R, Baumgartner H, Bleiziffer S, Borger Michael A, et al. Transcatheter or surgical treatment of aortic-valve stenosis. New England Journal of Medicine. 2024;**390**(17):1572-1583

[34] Talanas G, Laconi A, Kereiakes DJ, Merella P, Reardon MJ, Spano A, et al. Long-term outcomes of transcatheter vs surgical aortic valve replacement: Meta-analysis of randomized trials. Journal of the Society for Cardiovascular Angiography & Interventions. 2024;**3**(7)

[35] Liu Q, Mei J, Zhang H, Zhou W, Qiu K, Zhou Q, et al. A study of the novel SinoCrown system for transcatheter aortic valve implantation. EuroIntervention. 2023;**18**(17):1439-1441

[36] Skalidis I, Sayah N, Benamer H, Amabile N, Laforgia P, Champagne S, et al. Artificial intelligence and extended reality in TAVR: Current applications and challenges. Trends in Cardiovascular Medicine. 6 Aug 2025:ePub ahead of print. DOI: 10.1016/j.tcm.2025.08.002

[37] Reisman AM, Elmariah S. A review of "access to care" issues in aortic stenosis patients: A negative report card. Structural Heart. 2025;**9**(1):100351

Chapter 5

The Spectrum of Atrial Cardiomyopathy: Early Changes, Diagnostic Challenges, and Clinical Implications

Angelina Borizanova

Abstract

Atrial cardiomyopathy (AtCM) represents a progressive spectrum of electrical, mechanical, and structural atrial abnormalities that extend far beyond atrial fibrillation (AF) alone. Once considered passive reservoirs, the atria are now recognized as active contributors to cardiac performance, neurohormonal balance, and thromboembolic risk. Clinically, AtCM is highly relevant because it can drive complications such as AF progression, atrial failure, functional atrioventricular regurgitation, and even stroke or cognitive decline independent of AF. Practical staging frameworks incorporating imaging, electrophysiology, and biomarkers are beginning to guide risk stratification, yet routine application remains inconsistent. Advanced echocardiographic strain analysis, cardiac MRI for atrial fibrosis, and systematic ECG evaluation of P-wave morphology offer the valuable tools for early detection, but require broader clinical adoption. From a therapeutic standpoint, controlling modifiable risk factors such as hypertension, obesity, and diabetes is central to slowing disease progression. Early rhythm control strategies, including catheter ablation, may provide structural and functional benefit by preventing the vicious cycle of AF-driven remodelling. Furthermore, emerging insights into the role of epicardial adipose tissue, inflammation, and gut microbiota suggest novel upstream targets for preventive therapy. Current gaps in evidence, including optimal management of atrial functional regurgitation and thromboembolic risk in AtCM without AF, underscore the urgent need for prospective trials. This chapter emphasizes that AtCM is not merely an academic concept but a practical and clinically actionable entity. Recognizing its early manifestations, implementing multiparametric diagnostic strategies, and targeting systemic and atrial-specific mechanisms offer new opportunities to improve outcomes before irreversible atrial failure develops.

Keywords: atrial cardiomyopathy, atrial fibrillations, atrial failure, atrial functional mitral regurgitation, left atrial reservoir strain, atrial fibrosis

1. Introduction

Atrial cardiomyopathy is increasingly recognized as a distinct clinical entity that encompasses a wide range of atrial structural, electrical, and functional abnormalities. These changes may occur independently or in conjunction with AF, and often precede its onset. Unlike traditional views that regarded the atria as passive chambers, current understanding highlights their active role in cardiac performance, endocrine signalling, and thromboembolic risk.

This chapter aims to provide an in-depth overview of the spectrum of AtCM, with a focus on early-stage changes, diagnostic challenges, and their broader clinical implications. By exploring the multifactorial mechanisms behind atrial remodelling and dysfunction, we emphasize the importance of timely identification, risk stratification, and targeted intervention before the progression to irreversible atrial failure occurs.

2. Physiology of the atria

The atria play a crucial role in cardiovascular physiology, far beyond serving as passive chambers for blood transit. During the cardiac cycle, they function as reservoirs, collecting blood returning during ventricular systole, and as conduits, facilitating passive flow into the ventricles during early diastole. In late diastole, atrial contraction further enhances ventricular filling, contributing significantly to cardiac output—especially when ventricular compliance is reduced [1]. Classic pressure-volume analyses combined with Doppler echocardiography have elucidated these mechanical functions, demonstrating how the atria toggle between reservoir, conduit, and booster-pump roles to optimize ventricular loading [2, 3]. More recently, the atrium has also been recognized to exert a suction function, whereby rapid ventricular relaxation generates a pressure gradient that actively draws blood from the atrium into the ventricle, further enhancing early diastolic filling [4] as shown in **Figure 1**.

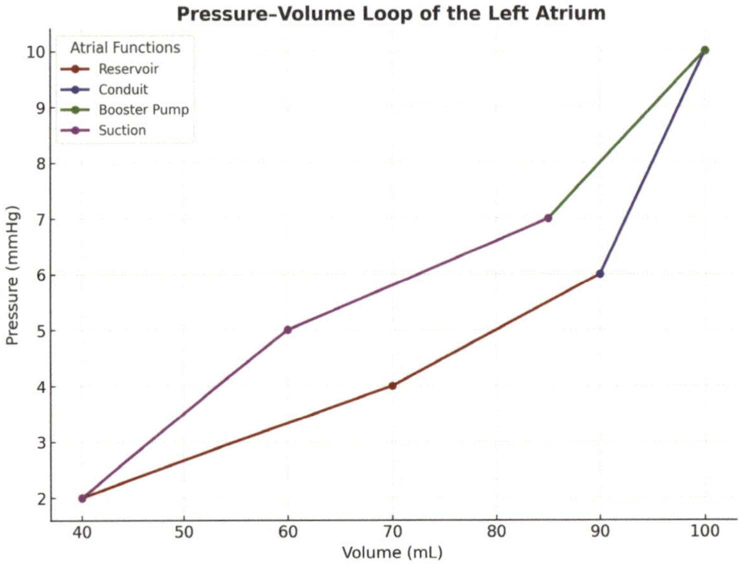

Figure 1.
Volume-pressure loop of the LA.

In addition to their mechanical functions, the atria are central to the heart's electrical activity. They house pacemaker cells in the sinoatrial node, which initiate cardiac rhythm, and components like the atrioventricular node, ensuring synchronized contraction—critical for efficient ventricular filling [5]. Moreover, the atrial myocardium has an important endocrine role—secreting atrial natriuretic peptide (ANP), which promotes natriuresis, vasodilation, and suppression of the renin-angiotensin-aldosterone system, thereby maintaining fluid and vascular balance [1].

3. Atrial cardiomyopathy and atrial failure: Definitions, clinical framework, and staging

Atrial cardiomyopathy is defined as a condition characterized by electrical and mechanical dysfunction of the atria, resulting from underlying pathological changes that can lead to atrial enlargement or fibrosis, with potential clinical consequences [6]. Diagnosis requires demonstration of electrical atrial dysfunction along with mechanical atrial dysfunction, atrial enlargement, or excessive fibrosis, helping to avoid over-diagnosis since multiple cardiac and systemic conditions can mimic atrial disruption [6].

AtCM may arise as a primary atrial disorder or secondary to existing ventricular or valvular disease. Similar to ventricular myopathy, AtCM exists along a spectrum of severity, and the combination of multiple atrial disease markers is associated with the higher risk of progression. Abnormalities may involve atrial geometry, wall structure, and function, typically assessed *via* cardiac imaging, electrophysiology, and biomarker evaluation [7, 8]. Surrogate markers such as advanced interatrial block, P-wave duration, and left atrial size have been linked to increased risk of AF, stroke, and thromboembolism, even in the absence of AF [9–12].

Early recognition of AtCM offers an opportunity to prevent atrial failure, the end-stage manifestation of progressive atrial structural, functional, and electrophysiological impairment. Atrial failure is clinically characterized by persistent AF or documented heart failure, often accompanied by dyspnoea, fatigue, and impaired

Stage	Description	Key features
Mild (subclinical) AtCM	Early-stage atrial remodelling	Detected by electrophysiology or imaging; no overt arrhythmia or significant mechanical dysfunction
Moderate (clinically manifest) AtCM	Evident atrial disease	Structural or mechanical abnormalities, elevated biomarkers (e.g. BNP, ANP), and/or manifest AF
Severe AtCM	Advanced atrial dysfunction or failure	LA ejection fraction $\leq$35%; severely impaired contractility (flow $\leq$20 cm/s in LAA or tissue strain); major interstitial alterations (fibrosis, fatty infiltration, amyloid, inflammation $\geq$35% LA wall volume); severe enlargement (LA diameter $\geq$5.0 cm, LA volume index $\geq$50 mL/m^2); long-standing persistent or permanent AF

Functional measurements (e.g. LAEF) are ideally obtained in sinus rhythm.
Prospective trials are needed to validate the staging system and cut-off values.
LA = left atrium; LAA = left atrial appendage.

Table 1.
Proposed staging system for AtCM [14].

quality of life attributable to atrial disease. Timely identification of AtCM allows for risk stratification and targeted management, including aggressive control of underlying risk factors and comorbidities [3, 6, 13].

A practical staging system for AtCM integrates imaging, electrophysiological measurements, and biomarkers, and distinguishes AtCM from AF, which can be both a consequence and a driver of atrial remodelling (**Table 1**) [14].

4. Left atrial cardiomyopathy: Multifactorial determinants

Left atrial cardiomyopathy (AtCM) represents complex and multifactorial conditions shaped by systemic, metabolic, behavioural, genetic, structural, and social determinants as shown in **Figure 2**. Aging promotes progressive atrial remodelling and fibrosis, predisposing to LA enlargement and functional decline [15]. Cardiometabolic diseases, including hypertension, obesity, type 2 diabetes, metabolic syndrome, metabolic dysfunction-associated fatty liver disease (MAFLD), and insulin resistance, impose chronic hemodynamic and metabolic stress that promotes left atrial remodelling, fibrosis, inflammation, endothelial dysfunction, and impaired diastolic function [16–18].

Among metabolic contributors, epicardial adipose tissue (EAT) has emerged as a pivotal player. EAT is metabolically active, directly interacting with cardiomyocytes; in obesity and diabetes, it releases pro-inflammatory mediators that foster atrial remodelling and fibrosis [19, 20]. Thus, metabolic dysregulation drives atrial disease through both cardiac and extracardiac mechanisms.

Emerging data highlight the role of the gut microbiota in atrial disease. Dysbiosis alters metabolite production and has been linked to cardiovascular conditions such as heart failure, hypertension, and obesity [21, 22]. Experimental and translational studies suggest that gut microbiota may promote atrial fibrosis and arrhythmogenesis, contributing to AF development [23, 24].

Behavioural factors, such as elevated alcohol consumption, independently impair LA reservoir and contractile functions and contribute to enlargement, particularly

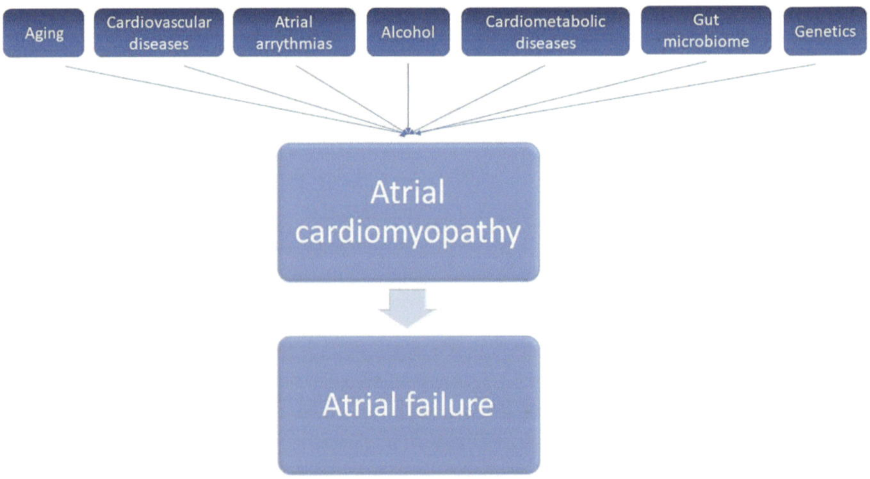

Figure 2.
Multifactorial determinants of atrial cardiomyopathy and atrial failure.

in high-risk populations [25]. Atrial fibrillation (AF) itself is both a cause and a consequence of remodelling, establishing a vicious cycle of structural and electrophysiological deterioration [26]. Heart failure with preserved or reduced ejection fraction (HFpEF/HFrEF) imposes sustained hemodynamic burden, diminishing atrial compliance and reserve [27]. Genetic predisposition modifies susceptibility to atrial remodelling and AF onset [28]. Social determinants of health, such as socioeconomic status, healthcare accessibility, and environmental stressors, also shape outcomes [29].

Finally, the concept of atrial cardiomyopathy underscores that LA pathology extends beyond chamber enlargement or dysfunction, encompassing cellular, structural, and electrophysiological alterations that remain incompletely defined [13]. Collectively, these insights highlight the need for an integrated, individualized approach to risk stratification, monitoring, and early intervention in LA disease to prevent progression to atrial failure.

5. Mechanistic basis of atrial cardiomyopathy

Atrial cardiomyopathy emerges from a complex interplay of genetic predisposition, protein aggregation, inflammatory pathways, gut-derived influences, oxidative stress, and adipose-mediated structural remodelling—factors that underpin the development and maintenance of atrial fibrillation (AF) [30]. Genetic factors play a pivotal role, particularly in early-onset AF, where rare variants in cardiomyopathy and arrhythmia genes significantly increase susceptibility and impact mortality [31, 32]. Despite advances in genetic testing, challenges remain in clinical implementation due to the complexity of gene variants and phenotypic expression [33].

Protein aggregation, notably amyloid deposition, contributes to atrial structural remodelling. Wild-type transthyretin amyloidosis is recognized as an underdiagnosed cause of heart failure with preserved ejection fraction, often accompanied by atrial dysfunction [34]. Amyloid infiltration in atrial tissue generates an arrhythmogenic substrate that promotes persistent AF [35]. Similarly, beta-amyloid pathology observed in Alzheimer's disease may affect cardiac tissue, suggesting a systemic proteinopathy contributing to atrial dysfunction [36].

Inflammatory mechanisms are integral to atrial remodelling. Activation of the cardiomyocyte NLRP3 inflammasome enhances inflammatory signalling, facilitating atrial arrhythmogenesis [37]. This pathway is amplified in conditions such as obesity, where inflammasome activation promotes AF susceptibility [38]. Emerging evidence also implicates gut microbiota dysbiosis in age-related AF through NLRP3-inflammasome mediated pathways, highlighting gut-derived influences on atrial pathophysiology [23]. Anti-inflammatory lipid mediators like Resolvin-D1 demonstrate the protective effects by preventing proarrhythmic remodelling in experimental models of right heart disease [39].

Oxidative stress contributes to atrial remodelling *via* reactive lipid species such as isolevuglandins that covalently modify proteins and exacerbate tissue injury [40]. Pharmacological scavengers targeting these reactive dicarbonyls show promise in mitigating atrial remodelling and arrhythmogenesis with the favourable safety profiles demonstrated in human studies [41].

Adipose tissue, particularly epicardial fat, is a source of inflammatory mediators that promote atrial fibrosis and conduction abnormalities. Increased epicardial fat volume correlates with AF severity and reduced success rates of catheter ablation [42].

Human epicardial adipose tissue secretes proinflammatory cytokines that contribute to the local inflammatory milieu, facilitating structural remodelling of the atria [43].

In summary, atrial cardiomyopathy is driven by a multifaceted network of genetic, proteotoxic, inflammatory, microbial, oxidative, and adipose tissue-mediated mechanisms. Understanding these interconnected pathways is critical for developing the targeted therapies to prevent and treat AtCM.

6. Complications of atrial cardiomyopathy

Atrial fibrillation (AF) is the most common manifestation of atrial cardiomyopathy (AtCM) and acts as an accelerator of the pathological process [6]. In some cases, it is difficult to determine which disturbance is primary—AF or AtCM [6, 30]. It is well established that AF leads to the development of atrial cardiomyopathy and progression to atrial failure (**Figure 3**).

Atrial failure resulting from supraventricular arrhythmias involves activation of neurohormonal pathways, including the renin-angiotensin-aldosterone system and vasoactive peptides, which may cause chamber dilation with impaired systolic and diastolic cardiac function. In this scenario, the left ventricular myocardium shows inflammation, histopathological changes in cardiomyocytes, and loss of normal structure, composition, and function. These changes are typical for tachycardia-induced cardiomyopathy [6].

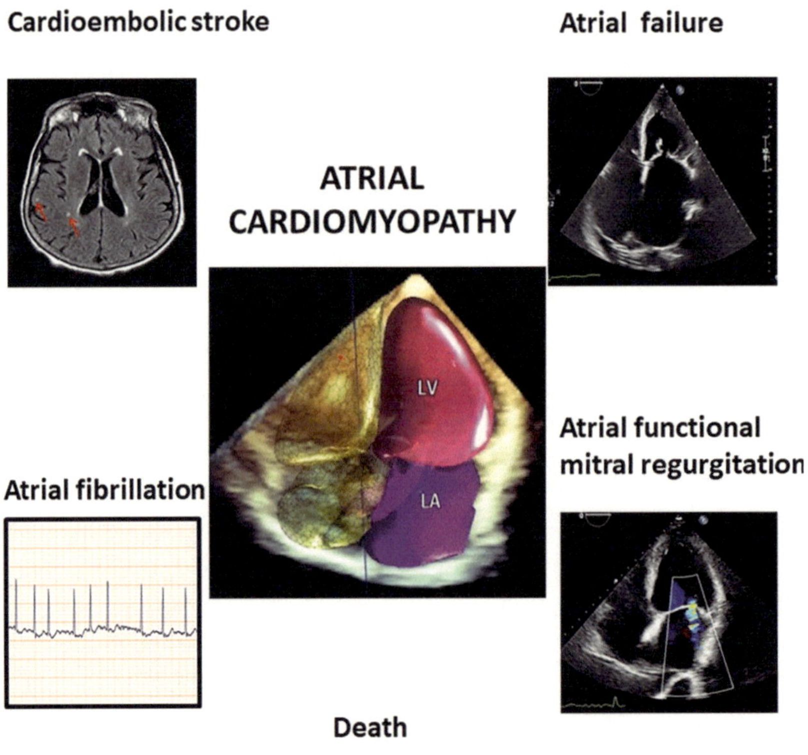

Figure 3.
Atrial cardiomyopathy complications.

Atrial functional regurgitations of the mitral and tricuspid valves are another complication of AtCM. Until recently, it was believed that atrial functional regurgitations were secondary to ventricular remodelling. However, in this context, ventricular geometry and function remain relatively preserved. The primary mechanism is annular dilation of the mitral and tricuspid valves, related to left and right atrial dilation, which results in poor leaflet coaptation and regurgitation. Additionally, increased left atrial pressure and reduced annular contraction contribute to impaired valve closure [6, 30]. A novel concept explaining atrioventricular functional regurgitations in patients with AF involves unfavourable annulus dynamics during fibrillation, including flattening and loss of the saddle shape [6].

In some patients presenting with *de novo* heart failure, disproportionate atrial cardiomyopathy relative to left ventricular function is observed, suggesting that left atrial dysfunction underlies heart failure manifestations. Atrial failure is likely an early "driver" of heart failure with preserved ejection fraction (HFpEF) and an important pathogenic risk factor [6].

Nevertheless, data regarding the thromboembolic potential of AtCM independent of AF and its association with stroke and dementia remain controversial [6].

7. Atrial cardiomyopathy diagnosis

Atrial cardiomyopathy (AtCM) represents a progressive spectrum, evolving from healthy atria to atrial failure. Diagnosing AtCM remains challenging due to its complex and multifaceted nature. To address this, simplified and clinically practical diagnostic criteria have been developed, which categorize AtCM into staged disease based on key features.

Diagnosis focuses on identifying electrical dysfunction alongside mechanical abnormalities, atrial enlargement, and/or evidence of fibrosis. This staged approach helps clinicians recognize and stratify AtCM progression, enabling earlier intervention to potentially halt or slow the transition toward atrial failure.

By breaking down AtCM into clearly defined stages, these criteria aim to improve clinical applicability, guide risk stratification, and support targeted management—especially in patients where controlling risk factors may prevent further atrial deterioration and its complications, such as atrial fibrillation and heart failure.

7.1 Electrocardiographic diagnosis of electrical atrial dysfunction in atrial cardiomyopathy

Electrocardiography (ECG) is the most commonly performed initial diagnostic test during a patient's first contact with a cardiologist. It plays a central role in identifying electrical abnormalities suggestive of AtCM, even before clinical AF manifests. P-wave abnormalities on a standard 12-lead ECG reflect altered interatrial conduction, atrial structure, and electrical function, and may signal early stages of AtCM.

A P-wave duration $\geq$120 ms on standard ECG or $\geq$ 150 ms on amplified ECG is a key marker of interatrial conduction delay and has been associated with increased risks of AF, stroke, cognitive impairment, and mortality [44–48]. Advanced interatrial block (IAB), defined as a P-wave $\geq$120 ms with biphasic (±) morphology in at least two inferior leads, reflects disrupted conduction through the Bachmann bundle and is closely linked to left atrial fibrosis and the development of AF—collectively termed Bayés syndrome [49–52].

Additional P-wave parameters such as low voltage (≤0.1 mV), abnormal axis (<0° or > 75°), terminal force in V1 (>40 mm·ms), and P-wave dispersion (>40 ms) have also been correlated with adverse cardiovascular outcomes and atrial remodelling [46, 48, 53–55]. To enhance clinical utility, a simplified ECG-based score has been proposed: a score of 1 for prolonged P-wave duration, 2 for advanced IAB without arrhythmia, and 3 or more for IAB with paroxysmal or persistent AF. This score helps stratify AtCM risk and guide preventive or therapeutic interventions [44, 46, 48, 54].

Given the ease of access, low cost, and early diagnostic value, systematic analysis of P-wave characteristics on ECG remains essential in recognizing electrical dysfunction in AtCM.

7.2 Mechanical dysfunction and fibrosis of the left atrium

Mechanical dysfunction of the LA is the central aspect of atrial cardiomyopathy, marked by impaired atrial function and structural remodelling. Accurate diagnosis is crucial for risk stratification and guiding treatment. Echocardiography, including 2D and 3D modalities, is the primary imaging method used due to its non-invasiveness, accessibility, and capacity for speckle-tracking strain analysis, which assesses atrial deformation and function [7, 55]. Cardiac magnetic resonance (CMR) provides advanced tissue characterization, enabling detection of fibrosis through late gadolinium enhancement (LGE), and offers highly reproducible measurements of LA volume and strain [56, 57]. Cardiac computed tomography (CCT) is primarily used for anatomical visualization and procedural planning but is less useful for functional assessment [58].

Left atrial reservoir strain (LASr) is the most established functional parameter, reflecting LA compliance and reservoir function during ventricular systole. Normal LASr averages around 39% in healthy adults, whereas values below 23–25% suggest impaired atrial mechanics and correlate with diastolic dysfunction and increased filling pressures [59–62]. Booster pump strain, representing active atrial contraction, shows abnormal thresholds below 5% for individuals aged 40–65 years and below 8% in those older than 65, indicating contractile impairment [63]. Additional functional markers include reduced LA emptying fraction—less than 48% on 2D and less than 43% on 3D echocardiography—signalling compromised mechanical performance [64].

Structurally, left atrial enlargement is gauged by the indexed left atrial volume (LAVi), a robust indicator of remodelling. Abnormal LAVi is defined as greater than 40 mL/m^2 by 2D echocardiography, with a higher cut-off of over 48 mL/m^2 for women older than 65 years [65–67]. Using 3D echocardiography, enlargement is identified above 41 mL/m^2, while CMR criteria set enlargement at volumes exceeding 60 mL/m^2 [68, 69]. These structural abnormalities are linked to an elevated risk of atrial fibrillation, stroke, heart failure hospitalizations, and mortality [70–72].

Atrial fibrosis is a hallmark of advanced atrial remodelling associated with arrhythmias and atrial failure. CMR with LGE imaging detects fibrotic tissue, with fibrosis affecting 10–15% or more of atrial tissue predicting higher arrhythmia and stroke risk [73–77]. However, CMR's use for fibrosis assessment remains largely investigational due to technical limitations and variability [78, 79]. Echocardiographic LASr inversely correlates with histological fibrosis, offering a valuable, non-invasive surrogate marker [80, 81].

Clinical evaluation for mechanical atrial dysfunction begins with 2D echocardiography, measuring LAVi and performing speckle-tracking strain analysis for LASr and booster strain. An LASr below 23–25% or an LAVi above 40 mL/m^2 (adjusted for age and sex) supports the diagnosis [61, 66]. Where available, 3D echocardiography or CMR can provide more accurate volumetric assessment and fibrosis evaluation, particularly in patients with atrial arrhythmias or prior stroke [57, 68, 75]. Integrating imaging findings with clinical and electrocardiographic data allows comprehensive identification of atrial cardiomyopathy and informs the prognosis and management strategies.

Early diagnosis of AtCM is essential for optimizing patient outcomes. Recent evidence highlights the diagnostic potential of combining advanced echocardiographic techniques, particularly left atrial strain analysis, with circulating biomarkers such as galectin-3 and high-sensitivity troponin I for the early detection of atrial remodelling in AF and AtCM [80]. This integrated, multimodal approach facilitates the identification of subclinical structural and functional changes in the left atrium at a stage when therapeutic intervention may be most effective. A more comprehensive approach to risk stratification and early treatment has the potential to improve long-term outcomes by intervening before overt atrial failure develops [6, 30]. Larger, prospective studies are now required to confirm these findings and to establish the standardized protocols for early diagnosis and personalized management of patients with AF and underlying atrial remodelling.

8. Prevention and treatment

Control of risk factors, especially modifiable ones, also ensures control over the development of atrial cardiomyopathy. Lifestyle changes, body weight control, physical activity, hypertension, and diabetes mellitus have proven benefits for cardiovascular health. AtCM is no exception. The role of renin-angiotensin-aldosterone system (RAAS) inhibitors and mineralocorticoid receptor antagonists in primary prevention remains controversial [82–84]. Recently, accumulating data support the use of cardiometabolic drugs as a means to influence cardiovascular complications. In a recently presented meta-analysis on the potential influence of cardiometabolic drugs on epicardial adipose tissue (EAT), the benefits of GLP-1 analogues for its control were demonstrated to be more significant compared to SGLT2 inhibitors. This effect was more noticeable among younger patients with significantly increased body mass index [4]. Further research is needed to provide information on the relationship between the modulation of EAT and the development of AtCM [85].

In patients with diabetes mellitus and atrial fibrillation (AF), treatment with SGLT2 inhibitors reduces AF episodes by 18% [86].

Treatment of AtCM is complex and depends on the complications that have occurred. In the presence of AF, rhythm control is certainly recommended to slow the progression of AtCM, as AF is known to accelerate the process. There is strong evidence for reverse atrial remodelling after maintenance of sinus rhythm [87–89].

In cases of functional atrial regurgitation, clear recommendations are still lacking. Undoubtedly, rhythm control is an important step since AF accelerates the process [90]. However, there is increasing evidence for successful transcatheter-based interventions in the treatment of functional atrial regurgitation [91].

The results of the ARCADIA trial did not confirm our expectations for anticoagulant therapy in patients with AtCM for the prevention of cryptogenic strokes [92]. In patients with an embolic stroke of undetermined source, rivaroxaban in the NAVIGATE-ESUS trial had no overall advantage over aspirin in reducing the recurrence of stroke or systemic embolism [93], except in patients with an LA diameter exceeding 46 mm [94].

According to current evidence, emerging clinical imperatives for AtCM emphasize the need for early and comprehensive approaches to detection, risk stratification, and management. The following recommendations are proposed:

1. Early detection: Implement multiparametric screening strategies, including atrial mechanical indices and biomarkers, to identify subclinical AtCM before the development of persistent arrhythmias or structural remodelling.

2. Risk stratification beyond atrial fibrillation (AF): Recognize AtCM as an arrhythmogenic and thrombogenic substrate independent of AF, warranting risk-based monitoring for complications such as atrial failure, stroke, and valvular dysfunction.

3. Bi-atrial assessment: Perform routine evaluation of both left and right atria, as remodelling frequently affects both chambers even in early stages.

4. Integration of advanced imaging: Utilize advanced imaging modalities such as cardiac MRI and echocardiography with speckle tracking and 3D imaging to assess atrial fibrosis and mechanical function where available.

5. Systemic risk factor control: Prioritize aggressive management of modifiable risk factors like obesity and hypertension to slow the progression of AtCM.

6. Longitudinal monitoring: Maintain close ambulatory follow-up, particularly in patients with early-stage AtCM or multiple cardiovascular risk factors, to enable timely therapeutic intervention.

7. Therapeutic reconsideration: Explore AtCM-specific therapeutic approaches, including upstream therapies and early rhythm control strategies even in the absence of sustained AF, aiming to prevent progression toward irreversible atrial failure.

9. Conclusion

Atrial cardiomyopathy is increasingly recognized as a distinct and complex clinical entity with significant implications for cardiovascular outcomes. It encompasses a spectrum of electrical, structural, and mechanical atrial abnormalities that may occur independently of atrial fibrillation AF, often preceding its onset. Despite growing awareness and emerging staging frameworks, AtCM remains underdiagnosed, and current diagnostic tools and treatment strategies are neither standardized nor specifically validated for this condition.

This chapter aimed to summarize the current evidence and provide a clinical foundation for recognizing and managing AtCM. However, major gaps persist in our understanding of its natural history, prognostic significance, and optimal therapeutic strategies. Dedicated prospective trials are urgently needed to refine diagnostic criteria, validate risk stratification models, and evaluate the targeted interventions.

Ultimately, viewing AtCM as more than a secondary consequence of AF or heart failure opens the door to earlier diagnosis, personalized management, and improved outcomes. Continued research and collaboration are essential to address this unmet clinical need.

Acknowledgements

Generative AI tools (including ChatGPT and GitHub Copilot) were used solely for language refinement and formatting assistance. All scientific content, interpretations, and references were prepared, verified, and approved by the author.

Conflict of interest

The author declare no conflict of interest.

Author details

Angelina Borizanova[1,2]

1 Department of Emergency Medicine, Medical University, Sofia, Bulgaria

2 Clinic of Cardiology, UMHAT "Tsaritsa Yoanna- ISUL", Sofia, Bulgaria

*Address all correspondence to: borizanowa@abv.bg

References

[1] Zhang Q, Wang S, Zhang H, Wang K, Li W, et al. Evaluation of left atrial function and the relationship between left atrial stiffness index and exercise capacity in hypertension-related heart failure with preserved ejection fraction. Frontiers in Cardiovascular Medicine. 2024;**11**:1501004. DOI: 10.3389/fcvm.2024.1501004

[2] Pagel PS, Kehl F, Gare M, Hettrick DA, Kersten JR, Warltier DC. Mechanical function of the left atrium: New insights based on analysis of pressure-volume relations and Doppler echocardiography. Anesthesiology. 2003;**98**(4):975-994. DOI: 10.1097/00000542-200304000-00027

[3] Kittipibul V, Laufer-Perl M, Balakumaran K, Costanzo MR, Marwick TH, et al. Atrial mechanics, atrial cardiomyopathy and impact of atrial interventions. Journal of Cardiac Failure. 2024;**30**(10):1355-1366. DOI: 10.1016/j.cardfail.2024.06.017

[4] Bhatt A, Flink L, Lu DY, Fang Q, Bibby D, Schiller NB. Exercise physiology of the left atrium: Quantity and timing of contribution to cardiac output. American Journal of Physiology. Heart and Circulatory Physiology. 2021;**320**(2):H575-H583. DOI: 10.1152/ajpheart.00402.2020. Epub 2020 Dec 4

[5] Hoit BD. Left atrial size and function: Role in prognosis. Journal of the American College of Cardiology. 2014;**63**(6):493-505. DOI: 10.1016/j.jacc.2013.10.055. Epub 2013 Nov 27

[6] Weerts J, Ţica O, Aranyo J, Basile C, Borizanova-Petkova A, et al. Atrial cardiomyopathy: From healthy atria to atrial failure. A clinical consensus statement of the Heart Failure Association of the ESC. European Journal of Heart Failure. 2025;**27**(11):2173-2194. DOI: 10.1002/ejhf.3782. Epub 2025 Aug 5

[7] Pathan F, D'Elia N, Nolan MT, Marwick TH, Negishi K. Normal ranges of left atrial strain by speckle-tracking echocardiography: A systematic review and meta-analysis. Journal of the American Society of Echocardiography. 2017;**30**:59-70.e8. DOI: 10.1016/j.echo.2016.09.007. Epub 2016 Oct 27

[8] Benjamin EJ, D'Agostino RB, Belanger AJ, Wolf PA, Levy D. Left atrial size and the risk of stroke and death. The Framingham heart study. Circulation. 1995;**92**(4):835-841. DOI: 10.1161/01.cir.92.4.835

[9] Martínez-Sellés M, Elosua R, Ibarrola M, et al. Advanced interatrial block and P-wave duration are associated with atrial fibrillation and stroke in older adults with heart disease: The BAYES registry. Europace. 2020;**22**:1001-1008. DOI: 10.1093/europace/euaa114

[10] Larsen BS, Kumarathurai P, Falkenberg J, Nielsen OW, Sajadieh A. Excessive atrial ectopy and short atrial runs increase the risk of stroke beyond incident atrial fibrillation. Journal of the American College of Cardiology. 2015;**66**(3):232-241. DOI: 10.1016/j.jacc.2015.05.018

[11] Bisbal F, Baranchuk A, Braunwald E, Bayés de Luna A, Bayés-Genís A. Atrial failure as a clinical entity: JACC review topic of the week. Journal of the American College of Cardiology. 2020;**75**(2):222-232. DOI: 10.1016/j.jacc.2019.11.013

[12] La Rosa G, Morillo CA, Quintanilla JG, Doltra A,

Mont L, et al. Practical approach for atrial cardiomyopathy characterization in patients with atrial fibrillation. Revista Española de Cardiología (Engl Ed). 2024;**77**(8):656-666. English, Spanish. DOI: 10.1016/j.rec.2024.02.009. Epub 2024 Feb 29

[13] Petzl AM, Deo R. Left atrial cardiomyopathy: A puzzling disease process short of an easy answer. Journal of the American Heart Association. 2024;**13**(7):e034268. DOI: 10.1161/JAHA.124.034268. Epub 2024 Mar 27

[14] Goette A, Corradi D, Dobrev D, Aguinaga L, Cabrera JA, et al. Atrial cardiomyopathy revisited-evolution of a concept: A clinical consensus statement of the European Heart Rhythm Association (EHRA) of the ESC, the Heart Rhythm Society (HRS), the Asian Pacific Heart Rhythm Society (APHRS), and the Latin American Heart Rhythm Society (LAHRS). Europace. 2024;**26**(9):euae204. DOI: 10.1093/europace/euae204. Erratum in: Europace. 2025 Oct 7;27(10):euaf248. DOI: 10.1093/europace/euaf248

[15] Abhayaratna WP, Fatema K, Barnes ME, et al. Left atrial size: Physiologic determinants and clinical applications. Journal of the American College of Cardiology. 2006;**47**(12):2357-2363. DOI: 10.1016/j.jacc.2006.02.048

[16] Markman TM, Habibi M, Venkatesh BA, Zareian M, Wu C, et al. Association of left atrial structure and function and incident cardiovascular disease in patients with diabetes mellitus: Results from multi-ethnic study of atherosclerosis (MESA). European Heart Journal Cardiovascular Imaging. 2017;**18**(10):1138-1144. DOI: 10.1093/ehjci/jew332. Erratum in: Eur Heart J Cardiovasc Imaging. 2017 May 1;18(8):848. DOI: 10.1093/ehjci/jex130

[17] Raisi-Estabragh Z, McCracken C, Condurache D, Aung N, Vargas JD, Naderi H, et al. Left atrial structure and function are associated with cardiovascular outcomes independent of left ventricular measures: A UK Biobank CMR study. European Heart Journal Cardiovascular Imaging. 2022;**23**(9):1191-1200. DOI: 10.1093/ehjci/jeab266. Erratum in: Eur Heart J Cardiovasc Imaging. 2022 Aug 22;23(9):e331. DOI: 10.1093/ehjci/jeac119

[18] Fatema K, Bailey KR, Petty GW, Meissner I, Osranek M, et al. Increased left atrial volume index: Potent biomarker for first-ever ischemic stroke. Mayo Clinic Proceedings. 2008;**83**(10):1107-1115. DOI: 10.4065/83.10.1107

[19] Vyas V, Blythe H, Wood EG, Sandhar B, Sarker SJ, et al. Obesity and diabetes are major risk factors for epicardial adipose tissue inflammation. JCI Insight. 2021;**6**(16):e145495. DOI: 10.1172/jci.insight.145495

[20] Poggi AL, Gaborit B, Schindler TH, Liberale L, Montecucco F, Carbone F. Epicardial fat and atrial fibrillation: The perils of atrial failure. Europace. 2022;**24**(8):1201-1212. DOI: 10.1093/europace/euac015

[21] Gawałko M, Agbaedeng TA, Saljic A, Müller DN, Wilck N, et al. Gut microbiota, dysbiosis and atrial fibrillation. Arrhythmogenic mechanisms and potential clinical implications. Cardiovascular Research. 2022;**118**(11):2415-2427. DOI: 10.1093/cvr/cvab292

[22] Spasova N, Somleva D, Krastev N, Ilieva R, Borizanova A, et al. Trimethylamine N-oxide, cardiovascular risk and vascular alterations in middle-aged patients with risk factors. Bioscience

Reports. 2024;**44**(5):BSR20232090. DOI: 10.1042/BSR20232090

[23] Zhang Y, Zhang S, Li B, Luo Y, Gong Y, Jin X, et al. Gut microbiota dysbiosis promotes age-related atrial fibrillation by lipopolysaccharide and glucose-induced activation of NLRP3-inflammasome. Cardiovascular Research. 2022;**118**(3):785-797. DOI: 10.1093/cvr/cvab114

[24] Dobrev D, Heijman J, Hiram R, Li N, Nattel S. Inflammatory signalling in atrial cardiomyocytes: A novel unifying principle in atrial fibrillation pathophysiology. Nature Reviews. Cardiology. 2023;**20**(3):145-167. DOI: 10.1038/s41569-022-00759-w. Epub 2022 Sep 15

[25] Alam AB, Toledo-Atucha E, Romaguera D, Alonso-Gómez AM, et al. Associations of alcohol consumption with left atrial morphology and function in a population at high cardiovascular risk. Journal of the American Heart Association. 2024;**13**(7):e031915. DOI: 10.1161/JAHA.123.031915. Epub 2024 Mar 27

[26] Nattel S, Burstein B, Dobrev D. Atrial remodeling and atrial fibrillation: Mechanisms and implications. Circulation. Arrhythmia and Electrophysiology. 2008;**1**(1):62-73. DOI: 10.1161/CIRCEP.107.754564

[27] Abbasi SA, Shah RV, McNulty SE, Hernandez AF, Semigran MJ, et al. Left atrial structure and function in heart failure with preserved ejection fraction: A RELAX substudy. PLoS One. 2016;**11**(11):e0164914. DOI: 10.1371/journal.pone.0164914

[28] Ellinor PT, Lunetta KL, Glazer NL, Pfeufer A, Alonso A, et al. Common variants in KCNN3 are associated with lone atrial fibrillation. Nature Genetics. 2010;**42**(3):240-244. DOI: 10.1038/ng.537. Epub 2010 Feb 21

[29] Gomez SL, Shariff-Marco S, DeRouen M, et al. The impact of neighborhood social and built environment factors across the cancer continuum: Current research, methodological considerations, and future directions. Cancer. 2015;**121**(14):2314-2330. DOI: 10.1002/cncr.29345. Epub 2015 Apr 6

[30] Goette A, Kalman JM, Aguinaga L, et al. Atrial cardiomyopathy revisited—Evolution of a concept: A clinical consensus statement of the European Heart Rhythm Association (EHRA) of the ESC, the Heart Rhythm Society (HRS), the Asian Pacific Heart Rhythm Society (APHRS), and the Latin American Heart Rhythm Society (LAHRS). Europace. 2024;**26**(9):euae204. DOI: 10.1093/europace/euae204. Erratum in: Europace. 2025 Oct 7;27(10):euaf248. doi: 10.1093/europace/euaf248

[31] Yoneda ZT, Anderson KC, Quintana JA, O'Neill MJ, Sims RA, et al. Early-onset atrial fibrillation and the prevalence of rare variants in cardiomyopathy and arrhythmia genes. JAMA Cardiology. 2021;**6**(12):1371-1379. DOI: 10.1001/jamacardio.2021.3370

[32] Yoneda ZT, Anderson KC, Ye F, Quintana JA, O'Neill MJ, Sims RA, et al. Mortality among patients with early-onset atrial fibrillation and rare variants in cardiomyopathy and arrhythmia genes. JAMA Cardiology. 2022;7(7):733-741. DOI: 10.1001/jamacardio.2022.0810

[33] Roberts JD, Chalazan B, Andrade JG, Macle L, Nattel S, Tadros R. Clinical genetic testing for atrial fibrillation: Are we there yet? The Canadian Journal of Cardiology. 2024;**40**(4):540-553.

DOI: 10.1016/j.cjca.2023.11.022. Epub 2024 Mar 28

[34] González-López E, Gallego-Delgado M, Guzzo-Merello G, de Haro-Del Moral FJ, Cobo-Marcos M, et al. Wild-type transthyretin amyloidosis as a cause of heart failure with preserved ejection fraction. European Heart Journal. 2015;**36**(38):2585-2594. DOI: 10.1093/eurheartj/ehv338. Epub 2015 Jul 28

[35] Röcken C, Peters B, Juenemann G, Saeger W, Klein HU, et al. Atrial amyloidosis: An arrhythmogenic substrate for persistent atrial fibrillation. Circulation. 2002;**106**(16):2091-2097. DOI: 10.1161/01.cir.0000034511.06350.df

[36] Troncone L, Luciani M, Coggins M, Wilker EH, Ho CY, et al. Aβ amyloid pathology affects the hearts of patients with Alzheimer's disease: Mind the heart. Journal of the American College of Cardiology. 2016;**68**(22):2395-2407. DOI: 10.1016/j.jacc.2016.08.073

[37] Yao C, Veleva T, Scott L Jr, Cao S, Li L, Chen G, et al. Enhanced cardiomyocyte NLRP3 inflammasome signaling promotes atrial fibrillation. Circulation. 2018;**138**(20):2227-2242. DOI: 10.1161/CIRCULATIONAHA.118.035202. Erratum in: Circulation. 2019 Apr 23;139(17):e889. doi: 10.1161/CIR.0000000000000694

[38] Scott L Jr, Fender AC, Saljic A, Li L, Chen X, Wang X, et al. NLRP3 inflammasome is a key driver of obesity-induced atrial arrhythmias. Cardiovascular Research. 2021;**117**(7):1746-1759. DOI: 10.1093/cvr/cvab024

[39] Hiram R, Xiong F, Naud P, Xiao J, Sirois M, Tanguay JF, et al. The inflammation-resolution promoting molecule resolvin-D1 prevents atrial proarrhythmic remodelling in experimental right heart disease. Cardiovascular Research. 2021;**117**(7):1776-1789. DOI: 10.1093/cvr/cvaa186

[40] Davies SS, May-Zhang LS, Boutaud O, Amarnath V, Kirabo A, Harrison DG. Isolevuglandins as mediators of disease and the development of dicarbonyl scavengers as pharmaceutical interventions. Pharmacology & Therapeutics. 2020;**205**:107418. DOI: 10.1016/j.pharmthera.2019.107418. Epub 2019 Oct 16

[41] Pitchford LM, Driver PM, Fuller JC Jr, Akers WS, Abumrad NN, et al. Safety, tolerability, and pharmacokinetics of repeated oral doses of 2-hydroxybenzylamine acetate in healthy volunteers: A double-blind, randomized, placebo-controlled clinical trial. BMC Pharmacology and Toxicology. 2020;**21**(1):3. DOI: 10.1186/s40360-020-0382-y

[42] Wong CX, Abed HS, Molaee P, Nelson AJ, Brooks AG, et al. Pericardial fat is associated with atrial fibrillation severity and ablation outcome. Journal of the American College of Cardiology. 2011;**57**(17):1745-1751. DOI: 10.1016/j.jacc.2010.11.045

[43] Mazurek T, Zhang L, Zalewski A, Mannion JD, Diehl JT, Arafat H, et al. Human epicardial adipose tissue is a source of inflammatory mediators. Circulation. 2003;**108**(20):2460-2466. DOI: 10.1161/01.CIR.0000099542.57313.C5. Epub 2003 Oct 27

[44] Chen LY, Ribeiro ALP, Platonov PG, Cygankiewicz I, Soliman EZ, et al. P wave parameters and indices: A critical appraisal of clinical utility, challenges, and

future research-A consensus document endorsed by the International Society of Electrocardiology and the International Society for Holter and Noninvasive Electrocardiology. Circulation. Arrhythmia and Electrophysiology. 2022;**15**(4):e010435. DOI: 10.1161/CIRCEP.121.010435. Epub 2022 Mar 25

[45] de Luna AB, Massó-van Roessel A, Robledo LAE. The diagnosis and clinical implications of interatrial block. European Cardiology. 2015;**10**(1):54-59. DOI: 10.15420/ecr.2015.10.01.54

[46] Jadidi A, Müller-Edenborn B, Chen J, Keyl C, Weber R, Allgeier J, et al. The duration of the amplified sinus-P-wave identifies presence of left atrial low voltage substrate and predicts outcome after pulmonary vein isolation in patients with persistent atrial fibrillation. JACC: Clinical Electrophysiology. 2018;**4**(4):531-543. DOI: 10.1016/j.jacep.2017.12.001. Epub 2018 Feb 3

[47] Bayés-de-Luna A, Bacharova L. New electrocardiographic aspects of the P wave: Its value in clinical cardiology. Annals of Noninvasive Electrocardiology. 2023;**28**(3):e13053. DOI: 10.1111/anec.13053. Epub 2023 Feb 24

[48] Nielsen JB, Kühl JT, Pietersen A, Graff C, Lind B, Struijk JJ, et al. P-wave duration and the risk of atrial fibrillation: Results from the Copenhagen ECG study. Heart Rhythm. 2015;**12**(9):1887-1895. DOI: 10.1016/j.hrthm.2015.04.026. Epub 2015 Apr 23

[49] Ariyarajah V, Apiyasawat S, Puri P, Spodick DH. Specific electrocardiographic markers of P-wave morphology in interatrial block. Journal of Electrocardiology. 2006;**39**(4):380-384. DOI: 10.1016/j.jelectrocard.2005.11.002. Epub 2006 Mar 9

[50] Power DA, Lampert J, Camaj A, Bienstock SW, Kocovic N, Bayes-Genis A, et al. Cardiovascular complications of interatrial conduction block: JACC state-of-the-art review. Journal of the American College of Cardiology. 2022;**79**(12):1199-1211. DOI: 10.1016/j.jacc.2022.01.030

[51] Baranchuk A, Torner P, de Luna AB. Bayés syndrome: What is it? Circulation. 2018;**137**(2):200-202. DOI: 10.1161/CIRCULATIONAHA.117.032333

[52] Koutalas E, Zagoridis K, Intzes S, Symeonidou M, Zagoridou N, Karagogos K, et al. P-wave duration and interatrial block as predictors of new-onset atrial fibrillation: A systematic review and meta-analysis. Europace. 2023;**25**(Suppl 1):euad122.623. DOI: 10.1093/europace/euad122.623

[53] Gutierrez A, Norby FL, Maheshwari A, Rooney MR, Gottesman RF, Mosley TH, et al. Association of abnormal P-wave indices with dementia and cognitive decline over 25 years: ARIC-NCS (the atherosclerosis risk in communities neurocognitive study). Journal of the American Heart Association. 2019;**8**(24):e014553. DOI: 10.1161/JAHA.119.014553. Epub 2019 Dec 13

[54] He J, Tse G, Korantzopoulos P, Letsas KP, Ali-Hasan-Al-Saegh S, Kamel H, et al. P-wave indices and risk of ischemic stroke: A systematic review and meta-analysis. Stroke. 2017;**48**(8):2066-2072. DOI: 10.1161/STROKEAHA.117.017293. Epub 2017 Jul 5

[55] Cameli M, Mandoli GE, Loiacono F, Sparla S, Iardino E, Mondillo S. Left atrial strain: A useful index in atrial fibrillation. International Journal of Cardiology. 2016;**220**:208-213. DOI: 10.1016/j.ijcard.2016.06.197. Epub 2016 Jun 28

[56] Habibi M, Samiei S, Ambale Venkatesh B, Opdahl A, et al. Cardiac

magnetic resonance-measured left atrial volume and function and incident atrial fibrillation: Results from MESA (multi-ethnic study of atherosclerosis). Circulation. Cardiovascular Imaging. 2016;**9**(8):10.1161/CIRCIMAGING.115.004299 e004299. DOI: 10.1161/CIRCIMAGING.115.004299

[57] Maceira AM, Cosín-Sales J, Roughton M, Prasad SK, Pennell DJ. Reference right atrial dimensions and volume estimation by steady state free precession cardiovascular magnetic resonance. Journal of Cardiovascular Magnetic Resonance. 2013;**15**(1):29. DOI: 10.1186/1532-429X-15-29

[58] Truong QA, Bamberg F, Mahabadi AA, Toepker M, Lee H, et al. Left atrial volume and index by multi-detector computed tomography: Comprehensive analysis from predictors of enlargement to predictive value for acute coronary syndrome (ROMICAT study). International Journal of Cardiology. 2011;**146**(2):171-176. DOI: 10.1016/j.ijcard.2009.06.029. Epub 2009 Jul 16

[59] Cameli M, Ciccone MM, Maiello M, Modesti PA, Muiesan ML, et al. Gruppo di Studio Ipertensione, Prevenzione e Riabilitazione, Società Italiana di Cardiologia. Speckle tracking analysis: A new tool for left atrial function analysis in systemic hypertension: An overview. Journal of Cardiovascular Medicine (Hagerstown, Md.). 2016;**17**(5):339-343. DOI: 10.2459/JCM.0000000000000073

[60] Morris DA, Takeuchi M, Krisper M, Köhncke C, Bekfani T, et al. Normal values and clinical relevance of left atrial myocardial function analysed by speckle-tracking echocardiography: Multicentre study. European Heart Journal Cardiovascular Imaging. 2015;**16**(4):364-372. DOI: 10.1093/ehjci/jeu219. Epub 2014 Nov 3

[61] O'Neill T, Kang P, Hagendorff A, Tayal B. The clinical applications of left atrial strain: A comprehensive review. Medicina (Kaunas, Lithuania). 2024;**60**(5):693. DOI: 10.3390/medicina60050693

[62] Singh A, Addetia K, Maffessanti F, Mor-Avi V, Lang RM. LA strain for categorization of LV diastolic dysfunction. JACC: Cardiovascular Imaging. 2017;**10**(7):735-743. DOI: 10.1016/j.jcmg.2016.08.014. Epub 2016 Dec 21

[63] Xu TY, Sun JP, Lee AP, Yang XS, Ji L, Zhang Z, et al. Left atrial function as assessed by speckle-tracking echocardiography in hypertension. Medicine (Baltimore). 2015;**94**(6):e526. DOI: 10.1097/MD.0000000000000526

[64] Lang RM, Badano LP, Mor-Avi V, Afilalo J, Armstrong A, Ernande L, et al. Recommendations for cardiac chamber quantification by echocardiography in adults: An update from the American Society of Echocardiography and the European Association of Cardiovascular Imaging. Journal of the American Society of Echocardiography. 2015;**28**(1):1-39. e14. DOI: 10.1016/j.echo.2014.10.003

[65] Moller JE, Hillis GS, Oh JK, Seward JB, Reeder GS, et al. Left atrial volume: A powerful predictor of survival after acute myocardial infarction. Circulation. 2003;**107**(17):2207-2212. DOI: 10.1161/01.CIR.0000066318.21784.43. Epub 2003 Apr 14

[66] Schönbauer R, Kammerlander AA, Duca F, Aschauer S, Koschutnik M, et al. Prognostic impact of left atrial function in heart failure with preserved ejection fraction in sinus rhythm vs. persistent atrial fibrillation. ESC Heart Failure. 2022;**9**(1):465-475. DOI: 10.1002/ehf2.13723. Epub 2021 Dec 5

[67] Badano LP, Miglioranza MH, Mihăilă S, Peluso D, Xhaxho J, et al. Left atrial volumes and function by three-dimensional echocardiography: Reference values, accuracy, reproducibility, and comparison with two-dimensional echocardiographic measurements. Circulation. Cardiovascular Imaging. 2016;**9**(7):e004229. DOI: 10.1161/CIRCIMAGING.115.004229

[68] Haykal R, Kassar A, Chamoun N, Akoum N. The left atrium in heart failure with preserved ejection fraction: What we know and what we do not know. Heart Rhythm O2. 2025;**6**(7):1028-1038. DOI: 10.1016/j.hroo.2025.04.007

[69] Melenovsky V, Hwang SJ, Redfield MM, Zakeri R, Lin G, Borlaug BA. Left atrial remodeling and function in advanced heart failure with preserved or reduced ejection fraction. Circulation. Heart Failure. 2015;**8**(2):295-303. DOI: 10.1161/CIRCHEARTFAILURE.114.001667. Epub 2015 Jan 15

[70] Tsang TS, Barnes ME, Gersh BJ, Takemoto Y, Rosales AG, Bailey KR, et al. Prediction of risk for first age-related cardiovascular events in an elderly population: The incremental value of echocardiography. Journal of the American College of Cardiology. 2003;**42**(7):1199-1205. DOI: 10.1016/s0735-1097(03)00943-4

[71] Leong DP, Dokainish H. Left atrial volume and function in patients with atrial fibrillation. Current Opinion in Cardiology. 2014;**29**(5):437-444. DOI: 10.1097/HCO.0000000000000088

[72] Burstein B, Nattel S. Atrial fibrosis: Mechanisms and clinical relevance in atrial fibrillation. Journal of the American College of Cardiology. 2008;**51**(8):802-809. DOI: 10.1016/j.jacc.2007.09.064

[73] Oakes RS, Badger TJ, Kholmovski EG, Akoum N, Burgon NS, Fish EN, et al. Detection and quantification of left atrial structural remodeling with delayed-enhancement magnetic resonance imaging in patients with atrial fibrillation. Circulation. 2009;**119**(13):1758-1767. DOI: 10.1161/CIRCULATIONAHA.108.811877. Epub 2009 Mar 23

[74] Marrouche NF, Wilber D, Hindricks G, Jais P, Akoum N, et al. Association of atrial tissue fibrosis identified by delayed enhancement MRI and atrial fibrillation catheter ablation: The DECAAF study. JAMA. 2014;**311**(5):498-506. DOI: 10.1001/jama.2014.3. Erratum in: JAMA. 2014 Nov 5;312(17):1805

[75] Zahid S, Cochet H, Boyle PM, Schwarz EL, Whyte KN, Vigmond EJ, et al. Patient-derived models link re-entrant driver localization in atrial fibrillation to fibrosis spatial pattern. Cardiovascular Research. 2016;**110**(3):443-454. DOI: 10.1093/cvr/cvw073. Epub 2016 Apr 7

[76] Kamel H, Okin PM, Elkind MS, Iadecola C. Atrial fibrillation and mechanisms of stroke: Time for a new model. Stroke. 2016;**47**(3):895-900. DOI: 10.1161/STROKEAHA.115.012004. Epub 2016 Jan 19

[77] Caixal G, Alarcón F, Althoff TF, Nuñez-Garcia M, Benito EM, et al. Accuracy of left atrial fibrosis detection with cardiac magnetic resonance: Correlation of late gadolinium enhancement with endocardial voltage and conduction velocity. Europace. 2021;**23**(3):380-388. DOI: 10.1093/europace/euaa313

[78] Javadi N, Bismee NN, Abbas MT, Scalia IG, Pereyra M, Baba Ali N, et al. Left atrial strain: State of the art and clinical implications. Journal of

Personalized Medicine. 2024;**14**(11):1093. DOI: 10.3390/jpm14111093

[79] Verheule S, Sato T, Everett T 4th, Engle SK, Otten D, Rubart-von der Lohe M, et al. Increased vulnerability to atrial fibrillation in transgenic mice with selective atrial fibrosis caused by overexpression of TGF-beta1. Circulation Research. 2004;**94**(11):1458-1465. DOI: 10.1161/01.RES.0000129579.59664.9d. Epub 2004 Apr 29

[80] Borizanova A, Kinova E, Koleva V, Tica O, Kalaydzhiev PR, Goudev A. Integrated advanced echocardiographic and biomarker approach for the early detection of atrial cardiomyopathy in middle-aged patients with atrial fibrillation. Cureus. 2025;**17**(7):e88642. DOI: 10.7759/cureus.88642

[81] Goette A, Schön N, Kirchhof P, Breithardt G, Fetsch T, et al. Angiotensin II-antagonist in paroxysmal atrial fibrillation (ANTIPAF) trial. Circulation. Arrhythmia and Electrophysiology. 2012;**5**(1):43-51. DOI: 10.1161/CIRCEP.111.965178. Epub 2011 Dec 7

[82] Neefs J, van den Berg NW, Limpens J, Berger WR, Boekholdt SM, Sanders P, et al. Aldosterone pathway blockade to prevent atrial fibrillation: A systematic review and meta-analysis. International Journal of Cardiology. 2017;**231**:155-161. DOI: 10.1016/j.ijcard.2016.12.029. Epub 2016 Dec 23

[83] Rienstra M, Hobbelt AH, Alings M, Tijssen JGP, Smit MD, et al. Targeted therapy of underlying conditions improves sinus rhythm maintenance in patients with persistent atrial fibrillation: Results of the RACE 3 trial. European Heart Journal. 2018;**39**(32):2987-2996. DOI: 10.1093/eurheartj/ehx739

[84] Myasoedova VA, Parisi V, Moschetta D, Valerio V, Conte M, et al. Efficacy of cardiometabolic drugs in reduction of epicardial adipose tissue: A systematic review and meta-analysis. Cardiovascular Diabetology. 2023;**22**(1):23. DOI: 10.1186/s12933-023-01738-2

[85] Zelniker TA, Bonaca MP, Furtado RHM, Mosenzon O, Kuder JF, et al. Effect of dapagliflozin on atrial fibrillation in patients with type 2 diabetes mellitus: Insights from the DECLARE-TIMI 58 trial. Circulation. 2020;**141**(15):1227-1234. DOI: 10.1161/CIRCULATIONAHA.119.044183. Epub 2020 Jan 27

[86] Yoshida K, Yui Y, Kimata A, Koda N, Kato J, et al. Troponin elevation after radiofrequency catheter ablation of atrial fibrillation: Relevance to AF substrate, procedural outcomes, and reverse structural remodeling. Heart Rhythm. 2014;**11**(8):1336-1342. DOI: 10.1016/j.hrthm.2014.04.015. Epub 2014 Apr 13

[87] Neefs J, Wesselink R, van den Berg NWE, de Jong JSSG, Piersma FR, van Boven WP, et al. Thoracoscopic surgical atrial fibrillation ablation in patients with an extremely enlarged left atrium. Journal of Interventional Cardiac Electrophysiology. 2022;**64**(2):469-478. DOI: 10.1007/s10840-021-01056-1. Epub 2021 Sep 16

[88] Pump A, Di Biase L, Price J, Mohanty P, Bai R, Santangeli P, et al. Efficacy of catheter ablation in nonparoxysmal atrial fibrillation patients with severe enlarged left atrium and its impact on left atrial structural remodeling. Journal of Cardiovascular Electrophysiology. 2013;**24**(11):1224-1231. DOI: 10.1111/jce.12253. Epub 2013 Sep 10

[89] Soulat-Dufour L, Lang S, Addetia K, Ederhy S, Adavane-Scheuble S, et al. Restoring sinus rhythm reverses cardiac

remodeling and reduces valvular regurgitation in patients with atrial fibrillation. Journal of the American College of Cardiology. 2022;**79**(10):951-961. DOI: 10.1016/j.jacc.2021.12.029

[90] Rottländer D, Hausleiter J, Schmitz T, Bufe A, Seyfarth M, et al. Impact of intraprocedural residual mitral regurgitation on long-term survival: The MITRA-PRO registry 3-year follow-up. JACC. Cardiovascular Interventions. 2025;**18**(3):403-405. DOI: 10.1016/j.jcin.2024.10.019. Epub 2025 Jan 8

[91] Kamel H, Longstreth WT Jr, Tirschwell DL, Kronmal RA, Marshall RS, et al. Apixaban to prevent recurrence after cryptogenic stroke in patients with atrial cardiopathy: The ARCADIA randomized clinical trial. JAMA. 2024;**331**(7):573-581. DOI: 10.1001/jama.2023.27188

[92] Hart RG, Sharma M, Mundl H, Kasner SE, Bangdiwala SI, et al. Rivaroxaban for stroke prevention after embolic stroke of undetermined source. The New England Journal of Medicine. 2018;**378**(23):2191-2201. DOI: 10.1056/NEJMoa1802686. Epub 2018 May 16

[93] Healey JS, Gladstone DJ, Swaminathan B, Eckstein J, Mundl H, et al. Recurrent stroke with rivaroxaban compared with aspirin according to predictors of atrial fibrillation: Secondary analysis of the NAVIGATE ESUS randomized clinical trial. JAMA Neurology. 2019;**76**(7):764-773. DOI: 10.1001/jamaneurol.2019.0617

[94] Borizanova A, Kinova E, Goudev A. Unmasking atrial cardiomyopathy in middle-aged patients with AF: A call for early detection. European Journal of Internal Medicine. 2025;**140**:106356. DOI: 10.1016/j.ejim.2025.05.021. Epub 2025 May 27